Can We Live Forever?

# Can We Live Forever?

## A Sociological and Moral Inquiry

BRYAN S. TURNER

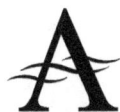

ANTHEM PRESS
LONDON · NEW YORK · DELHI

Anthem Press
An imprint of Wimbledon Publishing Company
*www.anthempress.com*

This edition first published in UK and USA 2009
by ANTHEM PRESS
75–76 Blackfriars Road, London SE1 8HA, UK
or PO Box 9779, London SW19 7ZG, UK
and
244 Madison Ave. #116, New York, NY 10016, USA

*British Library Cataloguing in Publication Data*
A catalogue record for this book is available from the British Library.

*Library of Congress Cataloging in Publication Data*

Turner, Bryan S.
   Can we live forever? : a sociological and moral inquiry/Bryan S. Turner.
      p. cm.
Includes bibliographical references and index.
ISBN-13: 978-1-84331-780-7 (hbk. : alk. paper)
ISBN-10: 1-84331-780-X (hardcover : alk. paper)
ISBN-13: 978-1-84331-794-4 (pbk. : alk. paper)
ISBN-10: 1-84331-794-X (pbk. : alk. paper) 1. Aging—Social aspects.
2. Longevity—Social aspects. 3. Longevity—Moral and ethical aspects. I. Title.
   HQ1061.T87 2009
   305.2601'12—dc22
                                    2009018402

ISBN-13: 978 1 84331 780 7 (Hbk)
ISBN-10: 1 84331 780 X (Hbk)

ISBN-13: 978 1 84331 794 4 (Pbk)
ISBN-10: 1 84331 794 X (Pbk)

1 3 5 7 9 10 8 6 4 2

*To the ageless Nguyen Kim Hoa*

# Contents

Acknowledgements    ix

Chapter One
Longevity and the Population Debate    1

Chapter Two
The Social Utopia of Human Perfection    27

Chapter Three
Ancient and Modern Techniques of Longevity    43

Chapter Four
The Political Economy of Ageing    69

Chapter Five
The Moral and Spiritual Character of Old Age    89

Chapter Six
Vulnerability and the Ethic of Care    107

Chapter Seven
Towards a New Paradigm of Ageing    125

Chapter Eight
The Aesthetics of Ageing    139

Bibliography    147

Index    157

# Acknowledgements

M any of the ideas in this book were originally developed as an aspect of the sociology of the body – a development in modern sociology that started in the early 1980s. My interest in ageing as a social process was first stimulated by Mike Featherstone and Mike Hepworth, whose ideas on the stages of life and the mid-life crisis first appeared in *Surviving Middle Age*. Mike Featherstone and I eventually came to edit the journal *Body & Society* where many of these issues were explored in the ensuing decade or so. Some of my criticism of the notion the body as 'socially constructed' was developed in conversations with Darin Weinberg at Cambridge University. Ideas about generational differences were originally developed with June Edmunds, with whom I eventually published *Generations, Culture and Society*. More recently I have published a series of articles with Alex Dumas, mainly on the political economy of ageing. I have also benefited from a visiting professorship at Flinders University and from debates with Anthony Elliott about the nature of social theory. Tom Cushman of Wellesley College has been an invaluable source of ideas about human rights and social theory. Tej Sood has been both patient and supportive in coaxing this book into existence for Anthem Press.

Some aspects of Chapter Six first appeared in my *Vulnerability and Human Rights* (Turner 2006) and some features of chapter eight were first examined in *The Body and Society* (Turner 2008). These arguments about vulnerability and the human body have been thoroughly revised in relation to this study of old age.

# Can We Live Forever?

# Chapter One

## Longevity and the Population Debate

### Introduction: Living or Surviving?

The quest for longevity appears to have been a recurrent theme in the history of human societies, because the possibility of extending life has persistently disturbed and provoked human consciousness. Awareness of our own finitude is a defining characteristic of what it is to be human and provides much of the foundation of religion, art and morality. In both fact and fiction, humans have long been pondering questions about longevity and happiness. Shakespeare's *King Lear*, in which the elderly king begins somewhat hastily and naively to surrender his sovereign powers to his daughters, may be a lesson about how not to become socially and politically irrelevant. At King Lear's court, the Fool warns the King not to grow old until he has grown wise. Similarly Jonathan Swift's *Gulliver's Travels*, in 1726, offered a humorous if also satirical and bitter account of the disillusion and depression suffered by the Immortals of the Kingdom of Luggnagg who were condemned to live forever. They have no memories of their youth and no hopes of any future release from the treadmill of life, thereby living their lives in a state of envy and moroseness. After his initial enthusiasm for the immortal Luggnaggians, Gulliver is informed that 'Envy and impotent Desires are their prevailing Passions' (Swift 2003, 196). Longevity had not trained them in superior virtues, but merely added to the existing list of mortal vices, and hence their immortality was farcical and pathetic.

Although the problems of death and survival have occupied human imagination throughout human history, the question – can we live forever? – has a distinctly modern resonance, since modern medicine holds out the actual rather than merely fantastic promise of survival without infirmity. At one level, the issue is simple: can we be old and healthy or is our own demise necessarily a depressing, debilitating and destructive experience? The optimistic answer looks towards technology and human creativity to solve the problems of ageing, the demographic imbalance and the crisis of resources. The optimists are in search of a medical utopia that can not only prolong life, but also remove its attendant disabilities. There is, needless to say, a long tradition of sceptical and critical responses to the promises of medical science and technology. René Dubos famously criticized modern medical utopias in his *Mirage of Health* (1959) in which he challenged the modern view that humans had achieved almost complete control over their environment and that they can control their own biological evolution and destiny. The pessimistic response to utopian thought is to argue either that technology cannot ultimately solve the problems of old age or, indeed, that technology actually compounds our difficulties. In the contemporary debate about ageing, the optimists are represented by people like the Cambridge biogerontologist Aubrey de Grey who, in *Ending Aging* (2008), treats ageing as an engineering problem and who advocates a plan to eradicate death from ageing through SENS – Strategies for Engineered Negligible Senescence. The pessimistic view he has dubbed the 'pro-aging trance', which induces the populace to accept ageing and its negative outcomes as natural and unavoidable. The pessimists are also dubbed the 'deathists'.

Rejuvenation sciences provide the solution to curing old age (as opposed to age-related diseases): 'Aging has been with us for a long time, despite our best efforts. The idea that it will be with us forever has ceased to be tenable, however, and the race is on to expedite its elimination' (de Grey 2004a, 2). The faith in the rejuvenation powers of medicine is often accompanied by anti-Luddite-inspired comments. Those who hold a negative perception on the life extension project are accused of possessing a conservative outlook, being unnecessarily reluctant to embrace social change and being constrained by rigid religious conceptions of the human lifespan, all of which restrict the so-called potential offered by anti-ageing technology. The quest to determine the pathological status of dying by old age in the light of recent scientific developments is a point that must be considered in depth if we are to understand where to set limits to scientific investments to extend life.

It is necessary to distinguish between different forms of life extension: a 'short life extension' that reflects demographic trends observed in the last centuries in the West and a 'long life extension' that, according to some biomedical scientists would enable humans to live well beyond the current maximum lifespan, unchanged in the last 100,000 years to around 125 years (Hayflick 2000). The former is the result of various social, political and medical developments, which, broadly speaking, are included in the conventional idea of 'the demographic transition'. The latter has resurfaced in the midst of the progress achieved in biomedical sciences, which attempt to alleviate, stop or reverse the ageing process (de Grey 2003). Life expectancy increased dramatically in the late nineteenth and twentieth centuries, but in the second half of the twentieth century it had reached a plateau in the majority of developed societies. If we consider men in the United Kingdom, the expectation of life at birth in 1901 was 45.5 years, but by 1991 this had increased dramatically to 73.2 years. However, subsequent demographic data show only a modest increase from 75.4 in 2001 to a projected 77.6 by 2020. This observed increase in the last century has had various significant consequences for society, and according to most conservative predictions, it will continue to produce important but often negative social, political and economic consequences over the next decades (such as the pension crisis, an elastic growth of public expenditure on health, uneven distribution of natural resources and changes in political representation). A sudden leap in longevity would inevitably create profound social disturbances. Although a radical change in life extension remains a futuristic goal, it does, however, have immediate repercussions on contemporary society, especially when issues pertaining to the prioritization of biomedical research and the concern for human rights are considered.

In December 1967 Professor Christiaan Barnard performed the first heart transplant operation at the Grote Schuur Hospital (Cape Town, South Africa) on a human patient. Experiments had previously been conducted on chimpanzees. In most of the early heart transplant operations, the patients died shortly afterwards. Barnard's patient, for example, died from pneumonia eighteen days after the operation. At the time, heart transplants were often regarded as mere medical gimmickry and they were condemned because they were expensive, high-technology solutions for a limited number of patients in a world where the mass of humanity, especially in Africa, lived relatively short lives with high levels of morbidity. Half a century later, we regard transplants of most human organs as routine medical procedures and modern medicine is now experimenting with replacement hearts that can be cultivated in the laboratory with modern genetic technologies. A heart transplant can be regarded as a technology for extending life and multiple transplants could be regarded as procedures necessary for living indefinitely.

Dr Barnard's heart transplant operation can be seen as proof of a project to treat the ageing body as a failing machine that was foreseen by an unusual partnership between the famous aeronaut Charles Lindbergh and the founder of tissue culture Dr Alexis Carrel, who, in developing experimental medicine, had grown human tissue outside the body. Having successfully flown across the Atlantic in 1927, Lindbergh wanted to harness experimental medicine to develop a cure for his sister-in-law who suffered from a defective mitral valve in her heart following an episode of rheumatic fever. Lindbergh's response to her impaired health was to approach the defective heart valve as one might respond to a defective oil pump in an aero-engine. When Lindbergh built a cooperative relationship with Carrel, the engineer and the experimental scientist dreamt of the possibility of one day removing the heart from sick patients and repairing it and then implanting the restored organ in the patient (Friedman 2007). The crucial aspect of Lindbergh's professional involvement with Carrel at the Experimental Surgery Division of the Rockefeller Institute for Medical Research (now The Rockefeller University) was Lindbergh's conclusion that death was simply the contingent outcome of failed bodily machines and that these mechanical failures were avoidable and unnecessary. Carrel and Lindbergh were successful in supporting living organs such as hearts and kidneys outside the body, but maintaining nerves proved to be a major obstacle. The idea that we can treat the ailing body as a defective machine has a long history, but it is only in recent years with the development of nanotechnology, for example, that the prospects of an engineering solution to ageing begins to gain greater feasibility and credibility. An engineering solution to the contingency of life can be regarded as the ultimate conclusion of Cartesianism in which the body as an object is merely an extension of the person (Turner 2008).

My assumption in writing this book is that today's gimmickry, or some version of it, for life extension will become routine in the next fifty years. Some version of Aubrey de Grey's 'engineering' solutions to the causes of ageing he has identified – cell depletion, cell excess, mutations of the chromosome, mitochondrial mutations, cellular debris, cross-linking – may also become commonplace procedures for prolonging life. Many of the other recommendations for delaying ageing – cosmetic surgery, vitamin supplements, dietary regimes, exercise, a modest consumption of red wine and so forth – are accepted without much debate. The more questionable 'solutions' such as massive calorie restriction, which are recommended by some pathologists – possibly as a solution for diabetes – may also become standard practice but in some modified form (Mason 2006). Perhaps an even more reliable and sophisticated version of cryonics – freezing whole bodies for some future restoration – might become part of mainstream medical technology.

My argument is that the technological changes are unstoppable and inevitable for three reasons. The first is the obvious motivation of economic profit. Prolonging life – whether in the conventional form of geriatric tourism, cosmetics, vitamin supplements, exercise routines or more exotic and unconventional techniques and regimes – is already big business and with an ageing population it will become bigger through an emerging retirement industry. Secondly, the desire of human beings to live longer is a more or less permanent feature of human society from ancient China to modern day California. Thirdly, there is a specific driving force that will be characteristic of the next three decades – the ageing of the Baby Boomer generation which has engaged in a lifetime of consumerism and social advancement and which is reluctant to relinquish these significant acquisitions of property and power. In the short term, we may expect life expectancy in the developed world to be well over one hundred years, but in the long term, life expectancy may simply keep increasing with new medical technologies. In this century, life expectancy could reach 150 years for such elite social groups. Profit, fame and desire will be sufficient to drive such technological experiments and medical advances.

Will the inevitable technological prolongation of life be a good thing? In this book, I start by making an economic assumption that scarcity is unavoidable and hence conflicts over resources are inescapable. Scarcity is not in my view a capitalist plot to make us compete for consumption items, and it is not a strategy of governments to control populations. It is a consequence of social change in a context of natural scarcity. Some natural resources – water, oil and timber – may simply be inadequate for human need. Extending life in a context of such natural scarcity must result in social conflict. Political scientists are already predicting future 'water wars', especially in Africa. Therefore, I explore some important negative consequences of this impending social and demographic transition, mainly in terms of social and political conflict. The prolongation of life by an Immortalist social movement will increase social conflict between generations and between the long-living elite and the impoverished majority. This elite will be the rich, primarily from the northern hemisphere, and the poor, primarily from the southern hemisphere, whose lifespan will actually decline, primarily from poverty, infectious diseases and low-intensity warfare over scarce resources. It may be that these medical technologies – such as stem cell therapies, organ transplants and cryonics – will become cheaper and more effective over time, and therefore available to a larger range of social groups. But we cannot anticipate a situation where these treatments will become universal. In the modern world, it is possible to treat AIDS/HIV with modern drugs, thereby controlling many of the unrelated conditions such as pneumonia that eventually kill the victims of this disease, but these drugs have not been available in much of Africa and Asia at an affordable price. If in some future world there is an effective anti-ageing drug, it is unlikely that this drug will be available in the war-torn areas of such a planet – the future equivalent of the Congo, Myanmar, Cambodia or Afghanistan.

There is however a more radical future – the unintended consequences of modern medical technology. In this book and elsewhere (Turner 2006a), I have argued that our humanity is defined by our vulnerability, which is in part a consequence of being an organism that grows old and is subject to ongoing morbidity. Vulnerability – from the Latin word for 'wound' – defines a shared world of risk, danger and death with which we can cope through a shared culture. Our collective institutions – law, government, religion and family – are social mechanisms that offer some respite from our vulnerability. Life-extension medicine promises to solve the problem of our vulnerability, but only and paradoxically by creating a posthuman world. The contemporary life-extension movement is driven by a profoundly individualist ideology that offers individual solutions but largely ignores many of the social consequences – generational conflict, the exhaustion of basic resources and massive regional inequalities. A cynic might argue that this situation is what we already have today. However, a significant increase in the Immortals in a world of declining fertility rates, political instability and existing scarcities would result, following the dystopian vision of Francis Fukuyama (Fukuyama 2002), in a posthuman world. Given my assumptions, I view this world with foreboding and alarm, but, because the Immortalist world view is what we might call a 'fix-it ideology', the Immortalist proposal is that we can live in a posthuman world provided we have the correct brain-enhancing antidepressant drugs. A postutopian existence could be tolerable with the appropriate pills to make us happy. In short, it is possible to build a social system based on eudemonism for the few and hardship for the many if we can secure an effective and efficient geriatric technology. As with most utopian and postutopian schemes, the argument comes down to an evaluation of technology. If the technological changes are inevitable, what justification for prolonging life might be ethically plausible? Is there a right to live forever? In this study, I put forward two visions of an extended life that might be justifiable. The political justification centres on the idea of a system of contributory rights and duties, and the second is aesthetic about the quality of life for individuals in which, rather than merely surviving, they are living life as a self-development.

## History and Life-Extending Technologies

Although modern medical technology has radically changed human life expectancy, in many respects the debate about ageing has not changed significantly. The interesting feature of the contemporary debate about ageing from the perspective of the history of social thought is that in many ways it parallels the debate between optimistic and pessimistic observers of modernization, human Enlightenment and the prospects of removing human suffering through the applications of Reason in the late eighteenth century.

The classical pessimistic view of the relationship between population, society and resources is associated with the demographic philosophy of Thomas Malthus, who was adamantly opposed to what he regarded as the utopian vision of writers such as William Godwin and the Marquis Condorcet. Godwin embraced the idea of human perfectibility, and similar reformist ideas that had been promoted by Condorcet in France. Against such visions of human development, Malthus, in *An Essay on the Principle of Population* in 1798, said that Condorcet and Godwin were idealists and failed to recognize that the laws of demography guaranteed a short life through famine and other catastrophes. Increasing wealth would increase fertility rates and, given more or less fixed resources such as cultivated land, the population would fall back as a result of pestilence and famine. The limitations of our life expectancy would not be overcome by science. This demographic constraint resulted from the fact that, while food and subsistence would grow arithmetically, population would geometrically, and hence natural resources, being limited, could not support a growth in population. Population growth could only be regulated by either preventive checks such as delayed marriage or by positive checks such as warfare, disease and famine. While preventive checks limited the birth rate, the positive checks ensured a high death rate. The result was to enforce a balance between population, land and the food supply.

The modern debate has similar characteristics between the optimists and the fatalists. The dominant literature on ageing until recent times has often tended to be both pessimistic and nostalgic. The classical example was Simone de Beauvoir's *Old Age* (1972) and in more recent times, intellectual biographies by philosophers like Norberto Bobbio in his *Old Age and Other Essays* (2001) have told the same story. In the conventional literature, there has been little to celebrate about age and ageing. Old age should be faced stoically since there are no alternatives to ageing and mortality.

This argument is an attempt at one level to develop further the insights of de Beauvoir. We could plausibly argue that the central questions of Western philosophy have been articulated around the mind-body dichotomy which we can describe in terms of the Platonic-Christian-Cartesian mind-body dualism in which spirit or mind or consciousness is always separated from and privileged over body (Shusterman 2008). This Western dichotomy was very different from the Asian understanding of the necessary connections between spirit and body. We might say that Asian cultures had a better understanding of embodiment, thereby rejecting simple dichotomies between spirit and flesh. Of course, not every branch of Western thought has been dualistic. The Socratic and Aristotelian view was that the care of the body is necessary for the life of philosophy and that, properly understood, virtue requires the discipline of the body. The Latin for 'virtue' was also connected with the idea of virility, thereby connecting virtuosity with virility. This mind-body split has a definite bearing on the problem of ageing because it raises, in another form, the problematic question of what is ageing? Is it only in the mind? Is it the decay of bodily functions and capacities, or should we regard it as an aspect of both?

Simone de Beauvoir is probably best known for her work on *The Second Sex* (1989) and, as a consequence, her work on *Old Age* (1972) has often neglected. In her critique of dominant views on sexual difference, she famously argued that the biological facts could not explain the hierarchy of the sexes, and that both men and women experienced the shame of the flesh in its pure, inactive, unjustified presence. Human nature is malleable, being shaped by history and circumstance. Social change cannot, however, be achieved through individual responses to our somatic condition, but only by collective social and political action. Somatic self-awareness, for de Beauvoir, can do nothing to improve our social circumstances. Her treatment of old age followed a similar logic. Ageing is not primarily a biological process but a social one in which, in a society that gives a special value to youth and youthfulness, ageing is brought about by the prejudicial gaze of our social contemporaries. What then is old age? She gives no clear answer except to say that it occurs because our vision is no longer refreshed by new projects. Old age is characterized by a lack of curiosity and by our need to cling to routines.

In the English-speaking world, popular interest in the causes of ageing was sparked off by Alex Comfort's *The Biology of Senescence* (1956). Public attention to the book was underlined by its republication in 1964 and 1979. Comfort was reacting to the theories of the German evolutionary theorist August Weismann (1834–1914) who was a strong supporter of Darwinian evolutionary science, but who rejected Darwin's notion of the inheritance of acquired characteristics. In 1883 in an essay on hereditary, Weismann (1891) explained that there is no mechanism by which changes in the external organs and tissues of an animal, resulting from environmental effects, could be conveyed to the reproductive organs and germ cells in them. The argument that germ-line cells contain information that passes to each generation independently of the somatic (body) cells came to be defined as the 'Weismann barrier'. He sought to prove this theory by cutting off the tails of twenty generations of mice to show that no mouse was subsequently ever born without a tail. While modern scientists no longer accept Weismann's barrier or his Germ Plasm theory, the distinction between the 'immortality' of the germ line and the mortality of the somatic line has become fundamental to modern biogerontological theories of ageing. From Weismann, contemporary evolutionary theory argues that genetic mutations that occur naturally by copying errors can also be produced by chemicals (mutagens). Some variations are more successful than others in reproductive terms, and through this indirect process and assortative mating, the genetic structure of a breeding group will change gradually.

Comfort became interested in Weismann because the distinction between germinal and somatic lines suggested a theory of ageing in contemporary science in terms of the 'disposable soma'. Weismann's evolutionary theory has been interpreted to mean that death in the individual occurs when a worn-out tissue cannot renew itself indefinitely. Weismann had said that the length of life depended on how many generations of somatic cells can succeed one another in the life of a single individual. Comfort was important because, following Weismann, he argued that ageing was fundamentally a biological problem, but he was critical of the extension of Weismann's cellular theory which had argued that 'worn-out individuals' are not valuable to the species because they stand in the way of sound individuals. In Weismann's framework, the death of such worn-out individuals is beneficial to the species and has an evolutionary significance. The breeding group gains maximum evolutionary advantage from the concentration of a large group of healthy individuals at one time. And by contrast, the survival of a large number of worn-out individuals brings no corresponding evolutionary advantage. Comfort complained that Weismann had simply assumed that the survival value of an individual must decline with the ageing process. Comfort proposed instead that senescence cannot have the evolutionary consequences suggested by Weismann, and that death and ageing had no beneficial relationship to evolution. Instead, ageing was a contingent or accidental outcome of selective processes shaping the life cycle of an organism up to the end of reproduction. What emerged from this earlier debate is that one cannot separate social and genetic processes too easily. To the question – why do individuals survive after their reproductive capacity has disappeared? – the answer, in part, is that social norms, prompting us to care for the elderly, explain why individuals can survive beyond their reproductive efficacy. To his credit, Weismann had clearly distinguished between biological and cultural evolution. As we shall see shortly, the argument now gets complicated regarding the interaction between cellular ageing, the greying of populations, and the social provision of healthcare to support the elderly.

But in order to engage effectively in this debate we need to establish some more precise notions about life expectation, prolongevity, ageing and old age. The possibility of 'living forever' has recently received a lot of attention partly as a consequence of the public recognition of the implications of stem cell research and related advances in medical science. Modern science has clearly brought about a whole new consciousness about age and ageing (Vincent 2006). However, in order to discuss these issues, we need to be clear about terminology. Probably one of the most useful historical accounts of these issues was developed by Gerald Gruman in his *A History of Ideas about the Prolongation of Life* (1966). Apparently Gruman (1966, 6) coined the term 'prolongevity' to mean 'the significant extension of life by human action'. In unpacking this definition, he argues that 'length of life' or 'longevity' has two meaning. The first is simply the number of years the average person may expect to live, and hence if the average age of death in the advanced countries is in the late 70s, we can refer to this as 'life expectancy'. The second meaning is 'lifespan' which refers to the longevity of the most long-lived human being. In modern times, the lifespan can reach over a hundred years, but lifespan has not, in fact, changed significantly. By contrast, life expectancy has risen dramatically with improvements in healthcare, diet and standards of living.

What then constitutes a 'significant' extension of life? Gruman divides scientific and philosophical opinion into two schools, namely those who believe that a major increase in lifespan is simply not possible, and those who believe it could be extended either greatly or indefinitely. The moderate debate is therefore essentially around the idea of prolonging the lifespan by medical intervention to bring about dramatic and significant increases. Furthermore, the medical goal of prolongevity must also be to reduce the disabilities, suffering and mental disorder that so often accompany ageing. Modern prolongevitism is quite definitely secular; the means to achieve prolongevity will come from secular biomedical sciences rather than from supernatural or magical means. The discourse of prolongevity is necessarily secular, according to Gruman, because Christian confidence in an afterlife has been shaken by the decline of religion as a general framework of belief and practice. Thus 'the modern era has been characterized by a marked decline of faith in supernatural salvation from death, i.e., immortality and resurrection by divine fiat' (Gruman 1966, 5). Gruman is essentially correct, but in my view, the theology of prolongevity will not go away so easily, because the promise of everlasting life in this world raises huge questions about the nature of humanity – questions that in many respects demand a theological answer.

## The Greying of Modern Societies

Peter Laslett (1915–2001) was a famous social historian of population change, especially of the modern history of Great Britain. In his historical demography, he shattered many myths about family history and structure, particularly in his *The World We have Lost* (1965). His empirical research in Northamptonshire and elsewhere in Great Britain demonstrated that in preindustrial society families were typically nuclear, composed of married parents and their children. Households were small and three-generation households were rare. His research destroyed the widely held view in sociology that the nuclear family was a modern product of industrialization and urbanization. He also showed that early modern English society was highly mobile in geographical terms and that each new generation residing in the same parish was uncommon. In his contribution to historical demography, he invented the term 'secular shift' to describe rising life expectancy in the century after the 1880s (Kertzer and Laslett 1995). This secular change was dramatic. If we take life expectancy at birth for men only in England and Wales, the increase was from 44.2 years in 1881 to 70.1 in 1991. Similar results for this period can be reported for other societies. For example, in the United States the increase was from 42.5 to 71.3; in Canada, from 43.5 to 73.0; in France, from 40.8 to 72; in Germany, from 35.6 to 71.8; and in Japan, from 42.4 to 75.5. The proportion of the population over 60 years of age during the secular shift rose in England and Wales from 7.4 per cent to 17.0 per cent; in the United States, from around 5.4 per cent to 15.9 per cent; in Canada, from 5.4 per cent to 11.3 per cent; in France, from 12.3 per cent to 16.6 per cent; in Germany, from 7.9 per cent to 16.7 per cent and in Japan there is no figure for the 1880s, but it was 12.9 per cent by the end of the twentieth century.

Let us focus in more depth on three cases: Japan, United States, and England and Wales. It is probably valuable to pause for a while over the Japanese case, because ageing in Japanese society is often quoted as an example of extremely rapid change, but the figures from Japan are also used to support arguments for dramatic policy changes to counteract the negative consequences of an ageing population. The population over the age of 65 will rise from its 1988 figure of 11.0 per cent to 23.6 per cent by 2021. Japanese women in particular are surviving in significant numbers into deep old age. In 2008 average life expectancy for Japanese women was 85 years and it is predicted to rise to 97 years by 2050. There are interesting regional variations, and it has been discovered that people in Okinawa have 600 people out of a population of 1.3 million who are centenarians – the highest density of centenarians in the world.

Similar outcomes have been found for the rate of ageing in the United States where the proportion of the population over 65 years rose from 12.4 per cent in 2000 to a projected 19.6 per cent in 2030. In absolute terms, the number of people over 80 years will rise from 35 million in 2000 to an estimated 71 million in 2030. There are, as in Japan, important regional and state differences. Florida had 19 per cent of its population over 65 in 2003 and it is projected to rise to 26 per cent by 2035. The percentage of the American population over 85 years was 0.1 per cent in 1900, 1.5 per cent in 2000 and an estimated 5 per cent by 2050.

In England and Wales, in 1948 7.2 per cent of the population was between 65 and 74 years and 2.9 per cent was between 75 and 84 years. In 2006 these figures were 8.2 per cent and 5.5 per cent. In absolute numbers those over 80 years have increased from 1,572,160 in 1981 to 2,749,507 in 2007. This age group is the fastest growing sector of the population.

We can also get a picture of ageing in these societies by looking at the statistics on centenarians. In 2007 the United States, with the largest population, unsurprisingly has 55,000 people of that age, while Japan has 30,000. In Okinawa there are five times more centenarians than in Japan itself. England and Wales had 9,000. It is estimated that by 2050 the United States will have 834,000 centenarians and the Social Security Administration has raised the prediction of life expectancy to 119 years of age. These increases in the number of centenarians are a reflection of the general rise in life expectancy and they illustrate significant improvements in hygiene, healthcare and medical advances.

These raw statistics of life expectancy are one aspect of the demographic transition that describes the historical shift from a period of high fertility and high mortality rates to a period of low fertility and low mortality. The causal factors that bring this transition about are much disputed, but broadly speaking, it was a consequence of improvements in the food supply, better public health provisions (clean water and sanitation) and eventually the impact of medical improvements (such as vaccination). The demographic transition also produced an epidemiological transition. Whereas in the past when most people died before they were old, the principal causes of death were infectious diseases; in the modern period the principal causes of death – cancer, heart disease and stroke – are among the elderly. It is this fact that causes most concern to governments, since disability increases rapidly among people over 65 years of age and the costs of caring for the elderly obviously have a major impact on health budgets. In 1990 around 1 per cent of the population in the United Kingdom was blind and 1 per cent deaf, but in the age group over 75 years 5 per cent were blind, 5 per cent deaf and almost 20 per cent were housebound. There has also been, throughout the developed world, a significant increase in people suffering from Alzheimer's disease and from Parkinson's disease. Although Parkinson's is not technically a fatal disease, it is associated with death from pneumonia, and in the United Kingdom it is identified as the thirteenth most common cause of death.

The Office of Health Economics in the United Kingdom has calculated that the costs to the National Health services will rise steeply with an ageing population. It has calculated that the per capita health cost at birth was £2,655 in 1999, whereas the cost per capita for the age group 45–64 years was £459. These costs increase sharply after 75 years. For the age group 75–84 it was £1684 and the costs over 84 years parallel the costs at birth, namely, £2639. The implication is that these outlays of public expenditure, with a significant increase in life extension, would increase exponentially. These data lend weight to the argument that increased healthcare could only be achieved through higher taxation or privatization or both. In the economic boom of the late twentieth century, many elderly people migrated to countries with a lower cost of living. For example, many Japanese retirees went to Thailand and Malaysia to reduce the economic burden on their families and some Asian societies now regard this strategy as an important aspect of economic development of the host society.

These changes in demography and epidemiology led James Fries (1980) to argue that in contemporary societies there is a compression of morbidity and mortality towards the end of life in which a temporary period of illness precedes death. In the past, morbidity, or the tendency to fall ill, occurred throughout the life course, whereas in the modern period it is compressed towards the end of life. This change results in 'the rectangularization of the survival curve' in which more and more people from a given generation survive into old age, when they die fairly rapidly from the principal degenerative diseases. Although this argument is useful in helping us to think about the characteristics of a greying population, Laslett (1995, 24) has questioned its accuracy by noting that, in fact, life expectancy shows no sign of faltering or declining. In short, the rectangular may never be actually described.

## The Scientific Debate

Medical interest in ageing goes back at least to writers such as Luigi Cornaro (1464–1566) who in his *Discorsi della Sobria* (*Discourses on the Temperate Life*) of 1558 argued in four discourses that his own longevity and happiness in old age were a consequence of temperance, exercise and a good diet. The body's finite supply of vital spirits could be husbanded by temperate practices of diet and exercise. His discourses, which were translated in 1903 and had an impact on American temperance ideas, are regarded as probably the earliest defence of a low-calorie diet. George Cheyne (1671–1743) took a similar view of the relationship between diet and healthy living in his *The Natural Method of Cureing* [sic] *the Diseases of the Body* in 1742. Despite the development of these medical regimens, the idea that the ageing of the human body is inevitable has been a basic presupposition of gerontology ever since. If ageing is an inevitable process of cellular degeneration, then the question about life extension does not arise, apart from mere fanciful speculation.

In most conventional gerontology, living a long life might in practical terms mean living a full life, according to some agreed cultural and social criteria, and achieving the average expectation of longevity by gender and social class. More recently however, there has been considerable speculation as to whether medical science could reverse the ageing process. Between the 1960s and 1980s, biologists expressed the view that normal cells had what was known as a 'replicative senescence', i.e., normal tissues can only divide a finite number of times before entering a natural stage of final quiescence. Cells were observed in vitro in a process of natural senescence, but eventually, experiments in vivo established an important distinction between normal and pathological cells in terms of cellular division. Pathological cells appeared paradoxically to have no such necessary limitation on replication, and therefore a process of 'immortalization' was the defining feature of a pathological cell line. Biologists concluded, therefore, by extrapolation, that finite division at the cellular level meant that the ageing of whole organisms was an inevitable process. These laboratory findings supported the view, shared by most religious and philosophical traditions, that human life had an intrinsic and predetermined limit, and that it was only through pathological developments that some cells might outsurvive the otherwise inescapable senescence of cellular life. Ageing was natural and normal, but it was also necessary if human societies are to avoid chronic overcrowding and the burden of an adverse dependency ratio.

This traditional framework of ageing was eventually disrupted by the discovery that human embryonic cells were capable of continuous division in laboratory conditions, where they showed no sign of any inevitable 'replicative crisis' or natural limitation. Certain nonpathological cells (or stem cells) were capable of indefinite division, and hence were in biological terms 'immortalized'. The cultivation of these cells as an experimental form of life has consequently challenged existing scientific assumptions about the distinctions between the normal and the pathological, and between life and death. Stem cell research begins to redefine the arena within which the body has renewable tissue, suggesting that the limits of biological growth are not immutable or inflexible. Research suggests that the human body has a surplus of stem cells capable of survival beyond the death of the organism. With these developments in microbiogerontology, the capacity of regenerative medicine to expand the 'natural' limits of life becomes a plausible prospect of medicine, also creating new economic opportunities in the application of life sciences. This new interpretation of replication locates human ageing within a shifting and unstable threshold between biological surplus and waste, or between obsolescence and renewal.

As we have seen, the modern theory of ageing depends on a distinction between the immortality of germ lines and somatic lines that takes us back to the legacy of August Weisman. He argued in terms of the germ plasm theory that inheritance only takes place through germ cells, namely the gametes such as sperm and egg cells. The other cells of the body or somatic cells do not exercise any agency in heredity. The 'Weismann barrier' describes the fact that information cannot pass from soma to germ plasm and thereby on to the next generation. Evolution is a trade-off between 'investments' in either soma or germ cells. Taking up Weismann's insights, contemporary scientists like Leonard Hayflick and Thomas Kirkwood remained dissatisfied with the way in which the relationship between individual ageing and evolution had been expressed in the debate surrounding Comfort's notion of senescence. Hayflick had revolutionized microbiology and cellular gerontology by discovering that normal human cells can only divide a finite number of times and it is this condition that determines senescence – a condition known as the 'Hayflick limit'. His research findings were popularized in *How and Why We Age* (Hayflick 1995) but interestingly, Hayflick has argued, in contrast to de Grey and others, that the goal of ageing research should not be to intervene in the ageing process. It should not be directed at increasing longevity but at the technical problem of discovering why an old cell is more vulnerable to pathology than a young cell. This question is important because scientific investment into the ageing process is infinitesimal when compared to funding for research on disease, and yet we know that the major causes of death – heart disease, stroke and cancer – are diseases of old age. Extending life expectancy has been achieved at the cost of increasing illness and disability in old age and, therefore, research on the lifespan should give way to research on why older cells are more vulnerable.

The result of this line of questioning is to separate the issue of evolutionary advantages to the breeding group from research on the vulnerability of cells. This issue has been clearly articulated in the research of Professor Kirkwood. Drawing on Weismann's distinction between germinal and somatic lines, Kirkwood interprets evolution as seeking a balance between the survival of germinal lines and somatic ones. The organism is the product of an investment in the somatic body to enhance successful reproduction and investment in the genetic lines to insure continuity of characteristics. Kirkwood's research has the effect of ruling out the notion of fixed genetic outcomes in ageing, because the issue of ageing is no longer the study of 'age-specific diseases', but the understanding of how somatic cells can carry out effective repair of cellular damage. He published his findings in various influential works such as *Time of Our Lives* (Kirkwood 1999) and *The End of Age* (2001).

What we might call the Kirkwood theory of ageing says: Ageing is the consequence of limited investments in somatic maintenance and repair, owing to competing priorities in reproductive investments; ageing is the outcome of damaged cells and tissues that have accumulated through the life course; a great variety of mechanisms contribute to the ageing process; the principal genes determining longevity are related to these maintenance functions such as antioxidant enzymes; longevity is programmed by the settings of genes relating to repair and maintenance; the maximum human lifespan is not fixed and determined, but malleable, for example, through the limitation of exposure to cellular damage. It is this proposition that the lifespan is malleable that has caused so much excitement among the optimistic Immortalists like de Grey, because it strongly suggested that we can engineer human longevity. It raises the further prospect that through the application of nanotechnology to the life sciences it may be possible, in principle, to devise a nanotechnological 'machine' that could enter the body to undertake microscopic repair of damaged cells. Thus the engineering dream of Lindbergh and Carrel would be realized.

The Kirkwood reinterpretation of the Weismann legacy also has important implications for the social and commercial exploitation of biogerontology. In an important article in *Body & Society*, Tiago Moreira and Paolo Palladino (2008, 37) point out that, following the Kirkwood approach, 'the business of biomedicine is to enhance the ability of the individual to imitate the immortal germinal line'. These scientific developments very specifically support anti-ageist social policies and hold out the promise of achieving a better fit between individual mortality and social functioning. Giving myself some licence, we might interpret the framework developed by Moreira and Palladino to suggest that human wisdom consists in recognizing that our biological constitution is merely a somatic vehicle for reproducing the genetic line. Furthermore, we might argue that the notion that we are simply constituted by the disposable soma is the ultimate definition of human vulnerability (Turner 2006a). The thrust of de Grey's position is that we can, in fact, delay the disposability of the soma by invasive and determined medical engineering, i.e., through rejuvenative medicine (de Grey 2004abcd and 2005abc).

The current popular interest surrounding the idea of significantly enhancing the human lifespan has penetrated various academic disciplines through the field of rejuvenation science, the science of preventing or slowing down age-related degeneration through interventions designed to extend one's healthy lifespan (de Grey 2004a, 1). For instance, the journal of *Rejuvenation Research*, which is indexed in most major scientific databases, is entirely dedicated to anti-ageing science, while the prestigious journal *Cell* has recently devoted an issue to the cellular mechanisms linked to the ageing process. In 2005 the Massachusetts Institute of Technology's

*Technological Review* featured a cover story on 'Living Forever' and in 2004 the *Scientific American* dedicated its second special issue to the sciences of staying young. In experimental research, genetic interventions aiming to extend the lifespan of various organisms (such as yeast, nematode, fruit fly and mouse) are now widely practiced in biological sciences (International Longevity Centre 2001). The healthcare industry is also participating through organizations such as the American Academy of Anti-Aging Medicine, which has an alleged membership of 11,500 physicians and scientists, and it aims 'to disseminate information concerning innovative science and research as well as treatment modalities designed to prolong the human lifespan' (American Academy for Anti-Aging Medicine 2005).

Scientific research seeking to prolong human life has generated a number of criticisms. Two main questions dominate the current debates on 'life extension': 'Can we live forever?' and 'Should we live forever?' The first question stems mainly from the field of biomedical sciences, concentrating on the feasibility of engineering a method capable of prolonging life, on the protection of consumers from quackery and on maintaining the credibility of biomedical science (Binstock 2003 and 2004; Hayflick 2005; Olshansky et al. 2004; Perls 2004). The second question is chiefly embedded in the fields of humanities and social sciences, being concerned with social and ethical issues (Cooper 2006; Fukuyama 2002; Kass 2002; Smart 2003; Vincent 2003). The works of Francis Fukuyama and Leon Kass have been particularly influential in recent years, both contesting the virtues of prolonging life beyond the 'normal' human life span.

The principal criticisms of the life extension science can be organized around two issues: the practical medical aspects of the project (for example, its feasibility and practicality) and social justice issues (for example, human rights questions). Because the life extension project implies the transformation of social institutions and changes in the allocation of resources, a sociological approach can contribute significantly to this debate. This book critically assesses the idea of life extension by evaluating the purpose of the scientific project, its implications for social justice and its repercussions on the sociology of ageing.

According to Gruman (1966, 75), most of the schools of 'prolongevism' before the seventeenth century were founded on religious beliefs and on primitivism, i.e., that prolongevity was possible since it was believed to have been achieved in the past. In biblical terms, human beings before their corruption by sin could expect to enjoy exceptionally long lives. During the Enlightenment, this view was replaced by the idea of scientific progress; prolongevitism and progress have thus evolved in tandem. With the growth of the authority of scientific values and assumptions in western societies (Schofer 1999), many frames of reference, such as religion, lost their legitimacy. Since the eighteenth century, the promise of science has not changed significantly; it has brought a message of hope, improvement and increased control over the body. The Human Genome Project, stem cell research and biomedical engineering have generated new hope of prolonging life, reducing morbidity and managing psychological illness in old age.

Because World Bank economists identified the ageing of the developed world as a significant threat to continuing global economic growth, there is considerable interest in the commercial possibilities of stem cell research as a feature of regenerative medicine. Companies operating in the Caribbean and Southeast Asia are already offering regenerative medicine as part of holiday packages, designed to alleviate the negative consequences of degenerative diseases such as multiple sclerosis or diabetes. Tourist locations around Phuket in Thailand, which are particularly popular among German tourists, offer a range of medical interventions to stave off ageing, alongside massage and casual sex. These social and medical transformations imply an interesting change from early to late modernity. In the early stages of capitalism, the social role of medical science was to improve healthcare, thereby making the working class healthy and efficient. The application of medical science was to produce an efficient labour force, but late capitalism does not need a large labour force at full employment, because technology has made labour more efficient. In this new biotechnological environment, disease is no longer a negative force in the economy, but on the contrary, an aspect of the factors of production. The economy can capitalize on disease by keeping people alive longer. It is thus very likely that the economic power of private corporations will have an important role in funding anti-ageing technology (Moody 2006).

The anti-ageing public discourse has emerged more intensely in the late twentieth century (Harber 2004). Drawing on the concept of governmentality (Foucault 2000), Katz (1996) has shown that through the pervasiveness of discursive practices in many areas of social life, ageing bodies have been constructed in negative terms; in the conjuncture of modernity and medicine, the old body became a social problem. The stigma of the ageing body, the dreaded fate of bodily finitude in secular thought (Mellor and Shilling 1993) and the sense of loss of control due to the erosion of physical capital (Dumas and Turner 2006), act as social vectors, which encourage public support for the life extension project.

The new approach to the science of ageing has resulted in a merger between the biomedicine business and governmentality, encouraging citizens to exercise responsibility for their own ageing and the dependency of their relatives. One implication of Kirkwood's science of ageing is that the diseases of the elderly are avoidable, being amenable to social and political interventions. Kirkwood had pointed out that ageing is primarily a disease peculiar to human societies, since animals in the wild rarely live long enough to experience ageing. Because 'death is a preventable and unnecessary event' (Moreira and Palladino 2008, 40), the new gerontology opens up huge commercial possibilities to improve lifestyle and diet to enhance the repair of the body and to delay its disposability.

## Justifying Long Life: Political and Aesthetic Criteria

This book is about the difference between surviving forever and living a satisfactory life that does not necessarily overburden the resources of society. But could we live creative lives through enhanced longevity and remain responsible to subsequent generations? Can we satisfy intergenerational justice? Part of my discussion of these issues, therefore, depends on a distinction between survival (can our organisms be sustained by modern technology?) and life (can we live as social beings in a cultural environment that sustains us?). In short, the question – can we live forever? – raises problems about nature (survival) and culture (life) that were central to Martin Heidegger's critical discussion of the relationships between Being, time and technology. The idea that we could live longer lives and live them more happily and with greater personal satisfaction rests ultimately on the notion that technological developments can solve the Malthusian problem (of inadequate resources in relation to population and land). Although nature has, so to speak, condemned me to a modest span of years with the prospect of disability and suffering in old age, technology in the modern shape of biomedical technologies can overcome what Malthus and the pessimists regarded as fixed laws of nature. The debate about nature and culture must address questions about ethics because the obvious criticism of the desire to survive forever is that it is a selfish desire in societies that have embraced 'possessive individualism' as a central doctrine. In such a society, the body is simply personal property and we have the expectation that with modern science we can sustain our bodies indefinitely, regardless of the cost to others.

In this study, therefore, I identify two frameworks or 'discourses' within which an extension of life might be justified. The first framework is political and legal. It says that we can have a right to life (partly as an extension of a right to healthcare). By implication rather than direct argument, it is assumed by de Grey and others that, as part of the right to healthcare, scientists should discover the causes of ageing in order to promote longer lives. However, a strong theory of rights requires us to find some duty that is correlated with the particular right. It is unclear what duty follows the right to an extension of life. On the basis of intergenerational justice, my right to a long life must be premised on my duty to give back resources to future generations. Indeed, a strict formulation of this argument would say that the resources that I consume in my lifetime should not reduce the opportunities of future generations to enjoy the same level of satisfaction in their lifetimes. This argument is based on an idea of justice as fairness (Rawls 1971). The length of my life should not undermine the opportunities of the next generation to live long and satisfying lives.

It is clearly very difficult to satisfy this criterion of fairness between generations. Governments, for example, attempt to create a 'level playing field' between generations by taxation on inherited wealth. The taxation of wealth is difficult because it is reasonable to argue that parents have a duty to pass on to their children a large part of their accumulated wealth. However, the idea of intergenerational equity is severely disturbed by the current trend towards increased longevity and it will be severely disrupted by prolongevity, i.e., by radical schemes for life extension. The idea of justice as fairness also has to cope with historical accident. For example, because I was born in 1945, my life was not severely disrupted by warfare, and postwar reconstruction offered me huge opportunities, whereas my father, who was born in 1910, sacrificed around six years of his life serving in the RAF in the Second World War. When and where we are born throws up contingent opportunities and risks that are highly unpredictable and very specific.

There is also a deeply puzzling economic issue about human life. In his *The Entropy Law and the Economic Process*, Nicholas Georgescu-Roegen (1971) claimed that waste is an unavoidable aspect of economic development and that human beings inevitably deplete natural resources and create environmental pollution with modernization. In an argument somewhat reminiscent of Malthus, he concluded that economic progress merely speeds up the inevitable exhaustion of the world's natural resources. His theory suggests that classical economics had neglected the problem of natural scarcity, believing that technology and entrepreneurship could solve the Malthusian problem of population growth in relation to fixed assets. Equally, the entropy law says that social conflict is inevitable because resources are scarce, humans degrade their environment and they must compete for limited space. Governments can attempt to reduce social conflict by extending social citizenship to all social classes, but the classical economics of Malthus and Ricardo avers that any reduction of conflict through, for example, income redistribution through progressive taxation will be modest and temporary. The life extension programme of modern Immortalists must necessarily increase waste and deplete the environment, and therefore will exacerbate social conflict. The rights discourse runs, therefore, into some fairly intractable problems. The second justification tends to be aesthetic.

One theme of this study is that while it is in principle possible to extend mere survival, the real issue is whether we can live creatively and successfully beyond mere survival. How can we cope with morbidity, boredom and the psychopathology of ageing? I suggest that, while medics have identified a process of biological waste at a cellular level, there is also a process that we might call 'social rusting' in which I accumulate a lot of social waste that makes it impossible to operate successfully in a constantly changing social and technical environment. In traditional societies, the old have wisdom because they understand tribal traditions. In the modern world, social obsolescence is a key problem in ageing. Happiness drugs are an unsatisfactory response to this problem since they merely mask these difficulties, creating the illusion that we are socially ageing successfully. Is there a drug for successful living? I argue, by analogy, that just as we become rigid in physical terms (physical vulnerability), we can also become mentally rigid. Following the argument of de Beauvoir that ageing is a loss of projects, I define ageing, therefore, as social and mental rigidity or inflexibility. We can only cope with social change successfully if we are constantly ready to redefine and refashion ourselves in order to avoid social irrelevance or social waste. This implies a certain psychological agility to counteract the boredom and spiritual apathy that normally attends old age eventually. Only in this sense would we have the right to live forever, since only through such persistent reconstruction could we continuously contribute to human culture, i.e., by remaining creative or lacking in rigidity.

This leads to the ethical nub of the debate about longevity. If I have a right to (try to) live forever, what duties might follow such a right? My answer is the duty of survival is very demanding – to try to add to the sum of human creativity in a manner that remains socially relevant and useful. Without such a duty, the right to live forever looks like human selfishness. Such an attitude may be justifiably regarded as a heroic view of ageing as self-construction and renewal, but in the interests of supporting the community rather than living parasitical upon it.

We might say that the aesthetic solution calls for a great deal of individual and social flexibility if we are to avoid or curtail the inflexibility of ageing. I am obviously and humorously referring to ageing as a form of social rusting in that getting old is like becoming a rusting bicycle. In human terms, ageing means mental rigidity and the accumulation of irrelevant knowledge that is of waste. If ageing is the accumulation of waste, we can at least take comfort from the fact that what we might call cultural or social ageing is not entirely confined to the elderly.

In conclusion, the question of *could* I live forever means both (1) is it physically possible for a human organism to survive indefinitely? and (2) *should* I live forever? This ethical question in turn implies the question: do I have a right to survive and, therefore, is there a duty to perform in order to justify living forever? With medical advances, one can imagine human rights issues becoming increasing central to ageing. The (United Nations) Universal Declaration of Human Rights says that we have a right to life; but is this a right to life lived indefinitely? – and at what cost to others? To avoid intergenerational inequality, we have an obligation to increase human resources, for example, human cultural resources (using culture here in its anthropological rather than aesthetic sense). In the final chapter on the 'aesthetics of ageing' I attempt to suggest a duty of creative living that is flexible but also responsible and thereby to combine the duty of citizens to manage scarce resources and the aesthetic calling of individuals to live creative lives. A general theory of successful ageing needs to combine the social duty of the conservation of resources with the possibility of creative living on the part of individuals. Living rather than surviving requires a robust and distinctive notion of life as a calling. The notion of a calling has strong religious connotations and hence, the problem is how to develop such a notion in a secular framework.

# Chapter Two
## The Social Utopia of Human Perfection

### Introduction: The Tithonus Fallacy

In his *The Living End*, Guy Brown (2008) effectively calls to mind a Greek myth – the story of Tithonus – to frame the debate about whether we can live longer lives *and* cure the geriatric diseases and disabilities that currently affect later life. In Greek mythology, Tithonus, a mortal, falls in love with Eos, the goddess of dawn. Realizing that Tithonus must die eventually, she asks Zeus to grant her lover immortality. Zeus, who is a jealous god, grants Eos's wish, but literally so. While Tithonus enjoys immortality, he does not also enjoy eternal youth. As Tithonus becomes old and decrepit, he also becomes demented and a burden. Driven to despair by his senile babbling, Eos turns her decaying lover into a cicada whose endless chirruping provides a parody of the babbling of the ageing Tithonus. The claim of contemporary immortalism is that medical science can ultimately grant us both immortality and eternal youth. By contrast, critics of medical science are allegedly committing the Tithonus fallacy of assuming that living forever is not desirable since senility will inevitably accompany longevity. Immortalists argue that people with the benefits of prolongevity can also be youthful, live fulfilling and happy lives and enjoy the benefits of continuous employment and social participation.

In the short term, these claims look utopian since, in old age, people, as a matter of fact, do accumulate disease and disability. In the long term, if we assume there can be a significant increase in longevity and youthfulness, then the question that confronts us is where would the social and economic resources come from to sustain such a population? In modern America, there is inadequate medical coverage and so it is unlikely that the costs of engineering longevity could only be sustained by the rich. In fact, the National Coalition of Health Care in its document 'Facts on Health Care Insurance' said that nearly 46 million Americans under the age of 65 years have inadequate health insurance. Furthermore, the medical costs of longevity could not be borne in poor countries and hence, the attempt to solve the Tithonus fallacy would only increase world inequality. Finally, while medical science may give us longer survival, can it give us longer life? These questions are closely connected with the idea that longer lives presuppose some radical transformation of society. Longevity presupposes social transformation and, hence, this issue is central to traditional political economy.

## Thomas Malthus, and Demographic Pessimism

Can we live forever? This simple question carries a lot of historical and ideological baggage with it. The obvious answer to the question is negative. In human history, despite rising life expectancy, very few humans live beyond one hundred fifteen years and, while there are now many more centenarians, we know that the final stages of life for the majority of people, even in developed societies, are accompanied by degrading and painful sickness and disability. The obvious retort to the question would be another question: Who would *want* to live forever? But realistic responses to this question may commit us too hurriedly and rapidly to a pessimistic vision of life as inevitably and necessarily fixed and limited. Medical optimists want us at least to consider the possibility that not only can life be extended, but it can be dramatically improved. Furthermore, the optimistic response invites us to separate two dimensions of this issue. The first is that there may be strong moral and social reasons to argue that we should not attempt to extend life indefinitely. The second is simply the factual dimension that wants to know in scientific terms whether life could be significantly extended by the application of modern medical knowledge and technology.

This debate in modern societies that involves both an awareness that many developed societies are experiencing the rapid ageing of their populations (e.g., Japan) and the realization that there are medical interventions that could in principle significantly extend human longevity tends to divide people into optimists and pessimists or into the so-called 'Immortalists' and 'deathists'. More profoundly, it divides people into those with a utopian vision of what is possible in modern societies and those with a dystopian vision who emphasize the negative and possibly inhuman consequences of significant prolongevity. In this study, I am particularly interested in the work of the Cambridge gerontologist Aubrey de Grey – who has been the most public advocate of life extension, of living forever – and his critics, who claim that his work is both dangerous and unscientific. I, too, have been (with my colleague Alex Dumas) a critic of the prolongevity argument of de Grey, mainly because it has, at least in the past, neglected the negative social consequences of extending the lifespan of the privileged social groups of the developed world. However, while one can easily criticize de Grey on these grounds, this negative view overlooks perhaps the more interesting question about a geriatric utopia. What visions are we fashioning for our own futures as human societies and can they be sustained?

In this discussion of the contemporary issues surrounding ageing populations, the rise in life expectancy and the quest to extend life more or less indefinitely by the application of medical technology, I am treating these contemporary debates over human ageing as simply the modern equivalent of the inquiry into human perfectability that was associated with the Enlightenment and the *philosophes* associated with the French Revolution. The modern argument that, with the applications of modern science, people could, in principle, live indefinitely and in relatively good health, implies quite clearly that the quality of human life can be subject to major improvement, indeed to medical perfectability. Life extension requires determination to set new standards of health and considerable research funding, but above all it implies the systematic application of medical reason to life. In the past, the optimists who advocated both human and social perfection included William Godwin, Mary Wollstonecraft and the Marquis de Condorcet. In the present, the optimistic camp includes the Methuselah Institute, the World Transhumanist Association, de Grey and SENS, the Cryonics Institute and individuals such as Ray Kurzweil. The original pessimists were essentially a group of economists who followed the arguments of David Ricardo, who believed that basic economic principles relating to natural scarcity meant that human life for the majority could not be significantly improved. As a result, Thomas Carlyle famously defined economics as a 'dismal science'. Perhaps the most influential negative response to the idea of both 'organic' and social perfectability was contained in Thomas Malthus's *An Essay on the Principle of Population* in 1798. The *Essay* immediately became the centre of a controversy in political economy and was followed by six editions during his lifetime (1766–1834). The first *Essay* was largely deductive and speculative, running to some 55,000 words. The second *Essay* in 1803 expanded the theory and included a great deal of illustrative data bringing the volume to 200,000 words (Petersen 1979). Further editions appeared in 1806, 1807, 1817 and 1826.

Malthus's arguments are relatively well known. In the first *Essay* he posited two 'fixed laws of nature', that food is necessary for existence and that sexual passion between the two sexes is more or less constant. The 'power' of population to increase is greater than the 'power' of earth to provide food. Population, if unchecked, will increase geometrically while subsistence can only increase arithmetrically. Human beings will, other things being equal, always generate more offspring than the means to sustain them in the long run. We need, therefore, to understand the checks and balances whereby population and resources can be properly arranged to avoid famine and overpopulation. In more elegant terms, in traditional societies, the relationship between resources (especially the food supply) and life expectancy was more or less regulated by a Malthusian logic. Given the sexual drive, the need for food and the declining yield of the soil, the increase in population would inevitably supersede the food supply. Population increase could either be controlled by what he called 'positive means' (such as famine, disease and war) or by 'preventive means' (such as vice, chastity and late marriage). Malthus was also aware of the issue of social class differences and noted that any attempt to improve the living conditions of the working class could not be sustained in the long term, because such reforms would increase the population, thereby reducing living standards by reducing the food supply.

Malthusianism is or has become identified with an essentially pessimistic view of the human condition since it does not allow for much in the way of human improvement. Technology will never solve the problem of the fixed quantity of land to provide food and improvements in farming technology will never quite meet the needs of human population. The sexual drive can be moderated by human institutions – including both celibacy and prostitution – but it cannot be ultimately controlled. Overpopulation will be a more or less permanent feature of human misery. But what has this got to do with ageing and prolongevity? Clearly, the Malthusian model assumes that human life cannot be significantly extended, because the elderly would be an additional burden on the resources of younger cohorts. An ageing population cannot be anything other than a demographic tax on the food supply and therefore the Malthusian model raises important issues about intergenerational justice, to which I shall return in subsequent chapters. A short life expectancy must be one aspect of the preventive means by which the balance between land and population can be sustained.

Malthus's *Essay* was not, so to speak, a piece of naïve demography. It was specifically addressed to those writers of his day whom he thought were hopelessly optimistic about the future of human beings. The optimists were the Marquis de Condorcet (1743–1794) who wrote his famous *Sketch for a Historical Picture of the Progress of the Human Mind* (1955), which was published posthumously in 1795, William Godwin in 1793 in *Enquiry Concerning Political Justice* (1946) and much later C. A. Stephens in *Natural Salvation* (1903). These were early optimistic proponents of prolongevity. These radical advocates of perfection were fundamentally influenced by a more general belief in scientific progress, and as a result they were more likely to perceive the shortness of the human lifespan as socially determined. They were committed to secular progress and were consequently hostile to traditional or religious views of the inherent and unalterable limitations on life. The moderate supporters of 'prolongevitism' were typically hygienists such as Luigi Cornaro, whose 'common sense' dietetics in his treatise on sobriety recommended lifestyle changes as the basis of an enhanced lifespan.

The late eighteenth century was a period of enormous optimism in which writers and political leaders such as Tom Paine and Thomas Jefferson welcomed revolutionary change, the fall of monarchies and the prospects of a universal recognition of the 'rights of man'. Paine believed that with the fall of monarchy, an age of peace and progress would begin. This political debate about revolutionary politics should be seen in the broader context of the Enlightenment in which Voltaire, Diderot and Leibniz looked optimistically towards the radical improvement of human society through the application of human reason. In England, the political debate about human rights, constitutionalism and human perfectability had been launched by the sermons and pamphlets of the Reverend Richard Price whose *A Discourse on the Love of our Country* (1927), which combined anti-Catholicism with an advocacy of basic political rights, was the occasion for Edmund Burke's hostility to the French Revolution in his *Reflections on the Revolution in France* (1955). Price had advocated the idea of citizenship of the world, universal benevolence and the doctrine of perfectability. Burke, by contrast, had argued that the 'rights of man' would result in social chaos. I want to start, however, with Condorcet and Malthus, because I think the modern problem is essentially one of political economy: If we live forever, can we be happy and will we deplete the environmental resources that will result in collective famine and misery? Is my happiness bought at the cost of the unhappiness of people in the Third World where life expectancy is now falling, not rising?

Marie Jean Antoine Nicolas de Caritat, Marquis de Condorcet was born in 1743 at Ribemont, Aisne in France, being descended from the ancient family of Caritat. His father died early, and his devoutly Catholic mother ensured that he was educated at the Jesuit Colleges of Rheims and de Navarre in Paris. A talented young mathematician, he soon came to the attention of Jean le Rond d'Alembert and Alexis Clairault. In 1765 he published a work on mathematics entitled *Essai sur le cacul integral*. In 1769 he was elected to the *Academie Royale des Sciences*. Condorcet is also famous as a consequence of his involvement in the French Revolution in 1789, in which he played a leading role. In 1791 he was elected as the Paris representative in the Legislative Assembly. His plans for the creation of a state education system were accepted and he drafted a new constitution for France. He advocated female suffrage, publishing the pamphlet entitled 'On the Admission of Women to the Rights of

Citizenship' in 1790. He also campaigned for the abolition of slavery. He did not support the execution of the French King, associating himself with the more moderate Girondist party. Because he opposed the so-called Montagnard Constitution, he was regarded as a traitor and a warrant was issued for his arrest. While in hiding, he wrote his *Sketch for a Historical Picture of the Progress of the Human Mind*, which was published posthumously in 1795. It is a major text of the French Enlightenment, showing the historical connection between the growth of science and the development of human rights. In March 1794 he attempted to escape from Paris, but he was arrested and imprisoned. He was found dead in his cell. The cause of his death has never been ascertained.

Who was Malthus? Born in 1766, the sixth of seven children, he entered Jesus College, Cambridge in 1784 and, becoming a deacon in the Church of England in 1789, he was ordained as a priest in 1791. The *Essay* was initially the product of a disagreement with his father Daniel Malthus, who supported the ideas of Godwin, Rousseau and Condorcet, believing that society was on a path to perfection. The application of science to human problems held out the promise that human and social improvements were almost inevitable. Against his father's optimism, Malthus attempted to demonstrate that the propensity of population to outstrip available land was an important and permanent check on social improvement and he saw no reason to believe that organic improvements were at all likely, even if human breeding could be modeled on animal breeding. Perhaps one obvious contradiction in Malthus's own position was how to reconcile this bleak picture of human existence with Christian theology. Malthus coped with this issue by arguing that humans are by nature lazy, but population pressure forces them to use their intelligence to correct the unintended consequences of the sexual drive.

Malthus starts volume two of the *Essay* with a painstaking criticism of both Godwin's and Condorcet's optimism. Malthus objects to the idea of 'the organic perfectibility of man' in Condorcet's work and asserts that the contradictions between the sexual drive and the limitations of the food supply can never be wholly overcome. It is worth, therefore, quoting his objections to Condorcet at some length:

From the improvement of medicine; from the use of more wholesome food and habitations; from a manner of living which will improve the strength

of the body by exercise, without impairing it by excess; from the
destruction of the two great causes of the degradation of man, misery and
too great riches; from the gradual removal of transmissible and contagious
disorders by the improvement of physical knowledge, rendered more
efficacious by the progress of reason and of social order; he infers, that
though man will not absolutely become immortal, yet the duration between
his birth and natural death will increase without ceasing, will have no
assignable term, and may properly be expressed by the word indefinite.

(Malthus 2004, 67)

The modern argument by those who argue in favour of indefinite
prolongevity is exactly the position of optimists like Condorcet for
whom the 'laws of nature' can be overcome by the application of
science and social reform. Malthus (2004, 68) admitted that changes
in climate and diet resulted in variations in life expectancy but he
argued that 'it may be fairly doubted whether there has been really
the smallest perceptible advance in the natural duration of human
life since first we had any authentic history of man.' However, for
him, to assume that at some future point in human history the laws
of nature would no longer operate was to abandon science in favour
of amusing ourselves with 'bewildering dreams and extravagant
fancies'. We will see in this study that de Grey and the optimists are
also accused of abandoning science in favour of utopian dreams.

## Criticisms of Malthusian Pessimism

History does not appear to have entirely supported the logic of this
Malthussian pessimism and most standard demographic textbooks
contain thoroughgoing criticisms of the Malthusian argument. For
example, in Britain, the invention of contraception in the 1820s, the
enhancement of the food supply through colonial expansion
and technical improvements in agricultural cultivation and
production controlled reproduction and expanded resources. With
improvements in nutrition, food supply and distribution, water
quality, public sanitation and housing, the death rate fell and the
increase in population was supported by technical improvements
in agriculture and the increase in cultivated land, partly through
technical improvements and partly through imperialism.
Eventually, the birth rate also declined as life expectancy rose with

the successful treatment of childhood illness such as whooping cough, and parents regulated their fertility. Throughout most of the modern world, there has been a dramatic decline in fertility.

With an increase in life expectancy, there is a critical problem surrounding ageing, but many assume that overpopulation is not the core issue. For many reformers, such as Amartya Sen and Martha Nussbaum, famine is a political issue that can be addressed by improving equality between social classes and by increasing the educational achievement of women. In many respects, these arguments also repeat the reformist philosophy of the Enlightenment period. In response to Burke's *Reflections*, Mary Wollstonecraft had supported Price's optimism in her *Vindication of the Rights of Woman* in 1792. The core of her defence of women's rights was the idea that through education, women could be lifted out of their servile and submissive social roles, and that motherhood and domestic slavery were not the only possibility for women. Modern reformers have also taken the view that to reduce female fertility, it is necessary to improve the level of literacy of females through education, thereby giving them the means to achieve greater equality.

Malthus's arguments have typically been the target of fairly critical, indeed violent responses. The literati rejected Malthus without qualification (Petersen 1979, 68–72). Lord Byron dismissed Malthus's ideas as crude economic speculation about marriage in which men were advised not to marry without cash. Shelley attacked Malthus because the social implications of Malthus's theories were conservative. Shelley argued that it was an injustice to ask the poor who were already suffering economic hardship to exercise restraint and responsibility. Coleridge thought Malthusianism was a cruel doctrine.

The standard criticisms of political economy appear to be convincing. Marx and Engels condemned the 'theory of increasing misery', since they could not accept the possibility that under communism this misery of the proletariat would continue. They, too, believed that through scientific management of the economy, these so-called 'laws of nature' would no longer apply. Joseph Schumpeter in his famous history of economic thought condemned Malthus (along with Ricardo) as a pessimist, noting that as the classical economists wrote their predictions of the tendency of the rate of profit to fall and the inevitability of low wages resulting from population pressures, Britain was on the eve of an economic boom.

In the modern debate about population pressures, Malthus and Malthusians are often characterized as right-wing ideologues employing the fear of overpopulation to convince people of the need for draconian measures to curb fertility. The scare about population pressures, according to his critics, has been used by neoliberal economists to argue that demography is being used to argue for cuts in welfare and pensions (Walker 1996). Certainly Malthus's views on working-class misery are typically quoted against him in this context.

However, at the time of the writing of this book in the early part of 2008, the international media were full of analyses of the end of the era of cheap food, the sudden increase in commodity prices generally and the global increase in the number of people who now find themselves below the poverty line. Some of these problems are probably short-term. They result from drought conditions in Australia and damaging floods in the American midwest; they are also partly the outcome of market speculation, and finally, a consequence of the increasing use of arable land to produce ethanol for fuel rather than food. The price increase may be moderated by the fact that farmers will be encouraged to plant more wheat, soya bean and rice in response to inflated commodity prices. However, the credit crunch that became increasingly evident around September and October of 2008 also suggests that the developed world will not invest in the underdeveloped world and that investment in green technology may shrink as governments attempt to secure energy supplies without close attention to environmental costs. If the decades of cheap money and easy credit have come to an end, then investment in longer-term projects to improve soil and agricultural production may be halted. These sharp increases in commodity prices at the beginning of the year were followed by a rapid decline in some commodity prices (such as oil) during the financial crisis and commodity crunch towards the end of 2008, indicating that aid to developing countries would be cut and investment programs in infrastructure would be severely limited. The prospects for health programs and social development are bleak for the immediate future. But are there more generic problems that point to the continuing relevance of Malthus?

Prior to the crisis of 2008, social scientists had assumed that the problem of the food supply was a thing of the past. One notable example of this attitude occurred in the otherwise brilliant essay of Daniel Bell in *Daedalus* (1987) in which he undertook a futurological inspection of 'the world and the United States in 2013'. Many of his assertions were realistic, such as his views on the rise of China as a world power. But his commentary on food is especially germane to this assessment of the Malthusian legacy. Bell spoke of a demographic time bomb, but this did not refer to the issue of the absolute growth of populations. In any case, he recognized that, in Europe, the population was already in decline. The real issue was the ratio of young people in the population as a whole. In Africa and Asia, the proportion of young people under fifteen years of age was around 40 per cent. The result would be 'demographic tidal waves sweeping the world' (Bell 1987, 16). By 2000, 70 per cent of the world's population would be concentrated in only eight countries: China, India, Indonesia, Brazil, Pakistan, Bangladesh, Nigeria and Mexico. These trends would create specific issues for the United States; for example, in its relationship to Mexico, would America have to absorb a large measure of Mexico's surplus youth population? But Bell did not see any problem in providing enough food to sustain an enlarged world population in the twenty-first century, observing that 'almost every country in the world is just about self-sufficient in food' and before 'the twentieth century, a famine was recorded almost every year somewhere in the world' but today they are rare (Bell 1987, 18).

This picture of world trends needs obviously to be modified. Firstly, the youth populations of many African societies have been devastated by HIV/AIDS and in many post-communist societies there are serious problems with venereal disease and addiction, as in Russia and increasingly in Vietnam. Secondly, Bell did not fully appreciate the steep ageing of populations in countries such as Japan, where the very future existence of a viable society is in question. Thirdly, there is a severe problem of rising commodities prices, especially food and oil, which, as we have noted, have driven many more people below the poverty line of one dollar a day for survival. Fourthly, there are severe pollution problems which very few countries have the political will to tackle. For example, when there were steep increases in the price of oil – rising in July 2008 to US $147 per barrel – truck drivers in Europe and fishermen in the Mediterranean went on strike, blocking roads and causing economic chaos. There were also food riots and urban crises in many societies, from Haiti to Egypt to the Philippines, over the price of rice, and Vietnam and Thailand stopped rice exports to guarantee a supply to their own people. Governments responded to these political pressures by measures that did not answer the long-term pollution problems caused by dependency on oil and the motorcar. On the contrary, they were often willing to look for measures to soften the blow of a spike in oil prices. We might imagine, therefore, that there is a continuum along which governments will select policies. At one end there is 'short termism', i.e., subsidies on oil prices or reduction of existing taxes or handouts to those groups that are adversely affected, such as taxi drivers. At the other end is the option of authoritarianism; for example, in Singapore people who protested against rising commodity prices were arrested because they did not have the correct permits to organize a meeting. A crisis in commodity prices in societies that have a weak tradition of democratic accountability will employ authoritarian measures to quell urban unrest among the surplus population of youth.

But there is another 'surplus population', namely, the elderly. There is a view among gerontologists that the elderly have rarely been able to form effective political lobby groups with the possible exception of the Gray Panthers in the United States. However, as the Baby Boomer generation approaches retirement and old age, will they be more inclined to form political movements? – they have, after all, been the major recipients of the benefits of the postwar economic boom in the West, and they have significant control of housing as a major asset. One issue behind the demand for prolongevity is the question of intergenerational responsibility. What, after all, is the driving force behind the quest for a longer life? The ideology of optimistic prolongevity is precisely the individualism that has been so important to the rise of consumer society in the postwar affluence, especially from around 1970 onward. We can, of course, trace the growth of a consumer society in the West to the 1930s when advertising became a significant feature of economic growth (Ewen 1976), but the development of a consumer ethic took a much more dramatic turn in the 1970s when the Baby Boomers were becoming established in the labour market. Cultural style became far more dominant in everyday life, especially for men, in the style magazines of the late twentieth century (Mort 1996). The quest for prolongevity – the answer to the question about indefinite life – is simply an aspect of the dominant ideology of consumption, individualism and happiness. In the late twentieth century, the combination of cheap money, credit and consumption presupposed, at least in societies like the United Kingdom and the United States, rising house prices. This strategy meant that personal savings could fall dramatically on the basis of rising house values. The crisis of 2008 is partly an adjustment to this imbalance between savings and expenditure, but this short-term crisis of credit has more ominous underpinnings – ageing populations, dissatisfied youth populations in the developing world, the dependence of the mature economies on labour migration, and rising commodity prices. This scenario is not exactly the Malthusian crisis of falling wages, overpopulation and a scarcity of land, but it does point to the disjuncture between the elderly rich (mainly in the northern hemisphere) and the young poor (mainly in the southern hemisphere).

However, the possibility of significantly extending the expectation of life in the affluent societies of the northern hemisphere through the application of medical research on stem cells has clear Malthusian implications for the world as a whole. The issues raised by Malthus suggest that there is no easy solution to the Tithonus fallacy, since increasing life expectancy in the affluent societies may occur while the underdeveloped world will suffer from declining incomes and diminishing resources. The bottom line of Malthus's pessimism is still with us, namely, that arable land is ultimately finite and technology has not discovered a fundamental remedy to this basic limitation. The ratio of people to arable land is a basic problem of the political economy of growth, and hence, the Immortalists have not really answered the question of scarcity, which is the basic economic issue.


## Conclusion: Baby Boomers and
## The Quest for Longevity

The Baby Boomers enjoyed a promising start to life with postwar reconstruction along Keynesian lines. However, this phase of British history around the construction of a welfare state came to a crashing halt with the first Thatcher administration of 1979–1983. Subsequently the 'Nanny State' became a target of much public criticism in the press. In academic life, British sociology increasingly became the study of consumer society with the decline of the old collectivist values that had been the social underpinning of the Labour Party and the welfare state. The Miner's Strike of 1984–1985 can be reasonably interpreted as the last working-class struggle to preserve the traditional values of Labour and the merits of collective action. Thatcherism ushered in not only a new political style, but a culture of consumption, celebrating mobility, greed and personal affluence. Hire purchase, credit cards and overdrafts were no longer a sign of moral decay, but essential contributions to the economy. Before the credit crunch of 2008, British high-street banks encouraged everybody to embrace personal loans, remortgage their homes and invest in overseas properties, typically as second homes in Spain and France.

The postwar generations who lived through the Cold War came to maturity in conditions of growing affluence and full employment. This period also saw the decline of the trade unions, and the erosion of social class as the most important marker of identity. While this generation was in fact always threatened by potential disaster, such as nuclear war during the Kennedy confrontation with Khrushchev, in retrospect Baby Boomers lived under conditions of relative peace. Compulsory military conscription, the ration book, barrack-room drill and the sheer cultural boredom of the 1950s had come to an end. The Beetles personified a new period in music and lifestyle when, at least briefly, British popular culture created a global lifestyle. Episodes such as the Suez crisis of 1956 demonstrated that Britain could no longer operate as a great power without American support and approval, and as a result, Britain subsequently withdrew from any further significant colonial adventures, including Mrs Thatcher's defence of British interests in the South Atlantic in the Falklands War in 1982. The pragmatism of Harold Macmillan set the standard of British foreign policy, allowing Britain to avoid the confrontations that dominated such colonial powers as France, Portugal and Belgium in the postwar period. Britain had no Dien Bien Phu.

Economic growth was characteristic of many parts of Europe and North America and in the economic boom from 1950 to the late 1970s, per capita growth in Europe rose from 1 per cent per annum to 4 per cent, and mass unemployment disappeared with unemployment rates falling from around 8 per cent to less than 2 per cent. Whereas Keynes had argued in his general economic theory that the problem of interwar economics was the 'stickiness' of money, i.e., people's reluctance to part with it, advertising helped people to feel comfortable with the constant translation of desire into actual purchase. Consumerism brought about a greater degree of social equality as holidays, homes, washing machines and motorcars became more widely affordable.

If consumerism does not need gods but only celebrity, it also tends to be a postheroic era, giving rise to what elsewhere I have called 'passive' generations (Edmunds and Turner 2002). If postwar student activism gave rise to the Campaign for Nuclear Disarmament (CND), anti-apartheid movements and eventually to the Events of 1968, the era of consumerism was eventually the era of Generation X. The apparent loss of heroic political activity was not confined to the West. In Eastern Europe, communist authorities were alarmed by the cynicism and disaffection of the postrevolutionary generations. The same disillusionment with postcolonial struggles has been also characteristic of Vietnam.

The ageing of the Baby Boomer generation brings to an end a significant and perhaps peculiar period of history. Having enjoyed wealth and social success, it is hardly surprising that this generation wants to retain its social influence through rejuvenative medicine. Their individualism and secularism are perfectly suited to a posthuman society where medical solutions that have individual benefits but no social merit are enthusiastically embraced. This is a generation that toward the end of its working life also experienced the late boom of the Reagan and Thatcher years. Its heroes have been the Rolling Stones who also show no inclination to leave the stage. Finally, it is a generation that is also well aware of the Tithonus Fallacy, because the real goal is to achieve both immortality and continuing youthfulness and health. The lifestyle of the Baby Boomers thus denies both ageing and death, embracing lifestyles that emphasize continuing activity, youthfulness and success.

# Chapter Three

## Ancient and Modern Techniques of Longevity

Many, I doubt not, will think that the attempting gravely to convert so absurd a paradox as the immortality of man on earth, or indeed, even the perfectibility of man and society, is a waste of time and words; and that such unfounded conjectures are best answered by neglect.

— Thomas Malthus (1798),
*An Essay on the Principle of Population*

### Introduction

In this chapter I compare and contrast the ancient quest for longevity through the search for an elixir of life with the growth of modern medical technologies that may assist the contemporary quest for longevity. The linking theme in this comparison is the centrality of technology to human culture. By 'technology' I mean not only machinery and equipment, but, more importantly, the techniques by which societies discipline the body with the aim of controlling either health or moral behaviour. These techniques of behaviour we can call, following Michel Foucault, 'the technologies of the self'.

Perhaps the key issue in this chapter is that, in thinking about old age and longevity, most societies have seen health and morality as being intimately connected. Hence, the technologies of the self typically seek to prolong life through promoting good health and at the same time embracing the notion that good health and longevity are consequences of moral probity. In short, most religious traditions have regarded longevity as the beneficial mark of a moral life. Perhaps the real break, therefore, between past generations and modern society is that our guides to good health have broken, or at least weakened, the link between moral behaviour and longevity. The result has been a profound secularization of our understanding of the life cycle and the connections between ethics and medicine. In the modern world, when we accept the idea that smoking cigarettes may seriously undermine our expectations of longevity, we do not argue that cigarette smoking is immoral. We merely recognize the fact that it can damage our lungs and heart, and probably much else.

However, one continuous theme in the history of the quest for longevity is that social elites, because they have the money, time and connections, have been at the forefront of social experimentation with medical techniques that are designed to promote longevity. The elites in most societies have sought out technologies and therapies that can help them live longer. In the past, knowledge about promoting longevity was often regarded as both powerful and dangerous, and therefore it was not to be shared with the masses. Knowledge of longevity was indeed often associated with the black arts and had to be practiced secretly and discretely.

One famous example of this quest for longevity, rejuvenation and potency comes from the life of the Irish poet W. B. Yeats. Through much of his adult life, Yeats feared the loss of artistic and sexual potency, which he believed came inevitably with old age. In the famous poem 'Sailing to Byzantium', Yeats described an elderly man as 'a paltry thing/A tattered coat upon a stick'. He was committed to the view that mind and body cannot be separated, and that the decline of one brought about the demise of the other (Pruit and Pruit 1983). Brooding upon his sexual decline and fearing the erosion of his poetic talent, Yeats became interested in the Steinach Operation, which he had read about in Trinity College Library Dublin. Eugen Steinach (1861–1944) was, by the 1920s, an internationally recognized medical specialist in the physiology of the sex glands and professor of biology at the University of Vienna.

He had come to the conclusion that hormone production was not only the crucial factor in sexual functioning but in well-being as a whole. The release of hormones into the human organism had the effect of rejuvenation. Discovering what he called the 'internal secretion' of the sex hormone and the 'external secretion' of spermatozoa from the testes, Steinbach experimented with various techniques that would enhance the production of hormones and the reduction of sperm. The most simple and effective was what we now call vasectomy. The operation, which was controversial, also had the beneficial side effect of functioning as a very effective contraceptive procedure and allegedly reduced high blood pressure and irritability, while increasing potency. In the 1920s over one hundred teachers and professors at the University of Vienna had the Steinach Operation. Sigmund Freud had it in 1923 to increase his potency in the treatment of his cancer.

On 6 April 1934 Yeats had the operation under the hands of Norman Haire, a Harley Street specialist who was also the President of the Sexual Reform Society and a strong advocate of the health benefits of sexual fulfilment. Yeats announced to a friend in the summer of 1934 that he had had the Steinach Operation with the overt intention of controlling his blood pressure, but the other benefits of the operation were apparently soon evident. Yeats, who was 68 years of age when he had his vasectomy, had at least four serious sexual liaisons in the years after the operation (Maddox 1999). His artistic productivity was also formidable and in the aftermath he published *A Full Moon in March* (1935), *New Poems* (1938) and *Last Poems* (1939).

Steinach's choice of the word 'rejuvenation' was probably dictated by commercial interests, and his method was certainly made popular by George Conners (1923), who brought out *Rejuvenation: How Steinach Makes People Young*. In retrospect, it appears, according to modern endocrinology, that vasectomy plays no part in hormone enhancement and that the Steinach Operation may have only had a placebo effect in raising the confidence of elderly men. Yeats's interest in Steinach was part of his more general interest in contemporary scientific developments. For example, he was particularly interested in eugenics, fearing the genetic decline of the elite and its political consequences. Yeats's confidence in science was, however, combined with a lifelong interest in the occult and astrology. As a young man, Yeats had joined the Hermetic Order of the Golden Dawn, a middle-class secret society combining rituals and beliefs from magic, the Kabbalah and Oriental wisdom. From 1917 onward, Yeats and his wife regularly attended seances in which Yeats was in communication with dead poets via a medium. His wife, Georgie Hyde-Lees, became his conduit to the spirits, and her capacity for Automatic Writing during trance-like experiences became an important source of guidance in his personal life. Yeats's quest for longevity cannot, therefore, be separated from his interests in magic and astrology, on the one hand, and eugenics and physiology on the other.

This association between the knowledge of the techniques of longevity and the magical arts arose because longevity may appear to challenge natural laws and the design of our Maker. The modern quest for longevity also raises questions about social justice, since only the elite will be able to afford the medical technologies that promise to keep us alive indefinitely. In this respect, while there is still an important issue about the distribution of resources in society, one might argue that the *ambition* to enjoy longevity has been democratized.

## Taoism and the Balanced Life

Perhaps the oldest medical tradition in the world emerged from Taoism in ancient China. While Taoism is difficult to define, it is best translated as 'the Way', involving the correct alignment of human life with nature. Its most important rituals were notably concerned with healing, funerals and the techniques necessary to obtain immortality. The identification of a distinct Taoist tradition is complicated by the fact that the three major religions of China – Taoism, Confucianism and Buddhism – have porous cultural boundaries, thereby borrowing promiscuously from each other. Within Taoism, there is a distinction made between the philosophical traditions that emerged during the Warring States Period (403–221 BCE) and its more religious manifestations at the end of the Han dynasty (206 BCE–220 CE). Central to Taoist teaching is the notion of the complementary relationships between *yin* and *yang*, and the notions of *ch'i*, the vital matter from which all things are made. Both notions have played an important part in Taoist thinking about longevity.

Comparing the Christian West and the East, Gruman (1966, 28) observed that in 'ancient and early-medieval China, a great philosophical–religious system, Taoism, was allied with prolongevitism. In the West, there was no development of comparable magnitude'. In the West, beliefs and practices relating to prolongevity were driven to the margins or even underground, whereas in China they occupied a central position. In Christianity, the aim was to survive in this world with the aspiration of eternal life in corporeal form in the next world after following a life of modesty and piety. By contrast, various strands of Taoist belief – the unity of nature, mysticism, quietism and primitivism – all contributed to the principle that life could be extended. Taoism developed a number of essential techniques that aimed to conserve energy and thereby promote longer life, namely respiratory, dietary, gymnastic, sexual and spiritual techniques. By these techniques, the sages who closely followed Tao could aspire to spiritual perfection, of which the ultimate sign was immortality.

From the third century BCE, individuals who were knowledgeable in the techniques for achieving immortality or *fangshi* ('the gentlemen with recipes') were being hired by the imperial courts to make their secrets available to the ruling class. These gentlemen were the official magicians to the court who performed many functions including exorcism and divination.

The fascination for an elixir of life motivated premodern science, especially in China. Belief in the existence of natural substances, or elixirs produced from them, that could prolong life was a significant aspect of Chinese medicine at least from the time of the Warring States. Because these substances included mercury, lead and arsenic, many alchemists suffered early deaths rather than enjoying longevity (Needham 1970). The preparation of these substances was costly and, therefore, the alchemists were typically members of the imperial court, providing services to the elite. The occupation of alchemist was thus precarious, since they were often accused of poisoning the emperor and hence were executed by the new incumbent. Needham raises the issue of where longevity could be spent. Confucianism did not have a clear idea of an individual soul and was in any case more interested in promoting social success and mobility in this world. Confucian scholars were reluctant to engage in any debate about personal survival. In orthodox, atheistic Buddhism, the notion of the persistence of the soul in an afterworld was wholly contrary to its original teaching. Taoism recognized a range of forms of existence, but after death they simply dispersed. The aim, therefore, of the medical elixir was to sustain existing life on this earth and to make it more enjoyable. It was therefore a distinctively secular medicine of this-worldly longevity.

The secular quest for life extension in China was not confined to experiments with elixirs. The Chinese notion of matter recognized the fluidity of material existence in which matter can become formless, only later to congeal and solidify. From these beliefs, there was the view that human life could be prolonged more or less indefinitely. Longevity (for men) depended on the production of semen and its retention in sexual intercourse. Taoist teaching on sexual relations involved correct adherence to appropriate seasons, time and rhythm. These views supported the idea of sexual intercourse as a therapeutic activity in which women supplied the yin components of life. A variety of sexual techniques were developed to prolong sexual intercourse and to delay orgasm thereby promoting longevity (Unschuld 1985). Given the theory of retaining the essence of matter, there was often a connection between 'black magic' and these life-enhancing techniques. Research on human remains in China suggests that cannibalism was practiced to acquire the power of other humans. The regenerative properties of human brains were especially favoured (van Straten 1983, 115). The brain and the spinal cord were thought to be the carriers of human life and therefore contained the basis for long life. On the one hand, there were techniques for retaining this vital energy, and on the other, techniques to expel impure matter from the body through gymnastics, diet and breathing. Both were aimed at preventing the slow loss of energy that characterizes normal ageing. In short, the techniques of longevity and the black arts both sprang from the same foundation, namely the concept of vital energy as the all-important substance for life.

It is from this period that we can find stories of the Immortals. These beings did not experience cold or hunger, they could enter fire or water without getting burnt or wet, and they could transform their old bodies into young ones. They could appear and disappear at will. These Immortals enjoyed a unique position in the hierarchy of beings, because they had fully realized the Tao and lived beyond the distractions of both terrestrial and celestial governments and their bureaucracies. Lu Dongbin, one of the group of Eight Immortals, created the Complete Perfection School and was the coauthor with Zhongli Quan of texts on alchemy. The Immortals were the apogee of Taoist thinking about the ideal harmonious relationship between nature and human beings.

One of the earliest medical texts is the Yellow Emperor's classic of internal medicine (*Huang Ti Nei Ching Su Wen*). The Yellow Lord or Yellow Emperor (Huang Ti) was part mythical emperor who belongs to the Age of Five Rulers lasting for some 647 years in the 'Legendary Period'. He is regarded as the founder of Chinese civilization and the first human ruler of the empire. More recent scholarship rejects the idea that this text can be attributed to the Yellow Emperor, regarding it instead as being written around 1000 BCE (Veith 1949). The actual origins of the text need not detain us. Suffice it to say that the text takes the form of a dialogue between Huang Ti and his minister Ch'I Po in which the emperor typically poses a question to which the minister gives an answer in the form of a discourse. The text contains the three themes that remained central to Taoist teaching and practice, namely, the Tao, yin/yang division and the theory of the elements.

The question of longevity occupied a central place in the account of internal medicine. Good health, which is the foundation of longevity, depends on behaviour towards the Tao. In fact longevity was a token of saintly character and an indication of effort to achieve complete adherence to the Way. The text refers to the ancient sages who lived long lives because they lived in harmony with heaven and earth, with the principles of yin and yang, and in accordance with the four seasons. Book 1 opens with the Emperor's observation that in ancient times the people lived to well over one hundred years, remaining active and free from disorders. The minister replied that the ancients understood the Tao, and organized their behaviour in terms of yin and yang. By contrast, in modern times 'people are not like this: they use wine as beverage and they adopt recklessness as usual behaviour' (Veith 1949, 97). The Emperor also asked Ch'iPo whether those who follow the right Way and get to one hundred years could beget children in their old age. The minister replied that 'Those who follow Tao, the Right Way, can escape old age and keep their body in perfect condition. Although they are old in years, they are still able to produce offspring.' (Veith 1949, 100)

Because longevity and health were identical, the process of ageing was necessarily a sign of disease. The medical canon had a clear and realistic picture of old age. Book Six of the Yellow Emperor's classic text describes ageing in an uncompromising fashion. 'When man grows old his bones become dry and brittle like straw, his flesh sags, the marrow within his bones disintegrates, and his movements deteriorate increasingly; when then (the pulse of the) kidneys is about to become noticeable, death will strike within one year, but if (the pulse of the kidneys) has become noticeable the allotted span is but one day'. The escape from this fate lay through strict devotion to the balanced life of the Way.

## Medieval Europe and the Pope's Body

The promise of eternal life was a central feature of the Nicene Creed and in societies with high mortality rates and short life expectancy, belief in an afterworld played a significant role in religious belief and practice. Christianity was itself originally a millenarian religious movement in which the expectation of a Second Coming and resurrection was a dominant religious theme of the early Church. The human body was a recurrent issue in medieval theological works including speculations about the physical survival of the Virgin Mary after death and about how devils possessed the human body. In Christian eschatology, there was a consensus that body and soul could not be separated without damage to human happiness and survival beyond life. Caroline Bynum (1991, 228) in her superb *Fragmentation and Redemption* notes that Aquinas, for example, argued that a 'full person does not exist until body (matter) is restored to its form at the end of time.' Of course the doctrine of physical resurrection raised acute conceptual difficulties for Christian theologians. Would, for example, the fingernails of an individual all be restored with resurrection? Could a person eaten by a dragon enjoy resurrection? The issue of the resurrected body was not, of course, merely an issue for theologians. It formed the basis of popular religious belief and practice with respect to the relics of saints and their miraculous healing of the laity. In these respects, Christianity has a decisively corporeal cosmology of the world.

In the Christian West, the search for an elixir of life was equally prevalent, at least among the elite. My account here depends heavily on the brilliant analysis of papal corporeality in *The Pope's Body* by Agostino Paravinci-Bagliani (2000) – originally published in 1994 as *Il corpo del Papa*. He shows how speculation about longevity was an important dimension of medieval theology, especially insofar as the spirituality of the pope was related to questions about the nature of longevity. Medieval popes had remarkably short lives and this fact was often taken as an indication of their profound spirituality. Nevertheless, popes were apparently as keen as the next man to extend life.

The vision of paradise in which the incorruptible body was everlasting was an important dimension of utopian thought. The imaginary world of Prester John – a world filled with abundance and wealth – was an object of considerable fascination during the rise of the papacy to supremacy, i.e., between the Concordat of Worms in 1122 and the Peace of Venice in 1177. For example, Lothar of Segni (later Innocent 111) wrote a commentary on old age in his *De miseria conditionis humane* in which he developed a mythical history in which, at the beginning of time, men lived for over nine hundred years, but with the onset of human decline, God, addressing Noah, created a new limit for men of one hundred and twenty years (Gen. 5:3), after which time, human life became shorter until the Psalms declared that the years of our life are merely threescore and ten. Life was characterized by its 'toil and trouble'. The Flood was a dividing point in human existence in which human decline is measured by the brevity of life. Lothar argued, however, that this brevity was important in squashing human delusions of the *prolongation vitae* and on this point he agreed fully with the Salerno medical school that the prolongation of life was not possible.

Thinking about age and ageing in this period was associated with the *De retardatione accidentum senectutis* – on delaying the misfortunes of old age – a work that was addressed either to the pope or the emperor. This work has occasionally but mistakenly been attributed to Roger Bacon (1214–1294), a Franciscan and leading Aristotelian. The attribution is related to the fact that Aristotle's *On Generation and Decay* itself played an important role in western medical doctrines about ageing, including the Salerno school, an important centre for translating Greek and Arabic texts. Salerno thus contributed to the latinization of Western medicine and produced such texts as the *Regimen sanitatis salernitanum*, which, in verse form, offered useful advice for healthy living such as diet, exercise and temperance (Porter 1997). While the Salerno school had rejected the idea of prolonging life, the *De retardatione* kept alive in medieval society the possibility of extending life through the discovery of appropriate ingredients.

Ageing was seen to be an effect of the decline of two humours (heat and moisture) that compose the human body in relation to two other humours (coldness and dryness). The secret of longevity was to discover those ingredients that retained heat and moisture while delaying the negative impact of cold and dry elements. The knowledge required to delay such developments was occult 'because he who possesses the secret of all their properties sooner or later transgresses the divine law; it follows that only the "wise in speculation" (*sapiens in speculatione*) and the "expert in the ways of things" (*expertus in operatione*) can derive "noble and sublime" profit from such substances' (Paravinci-Bagliani 2000, 203). The treatise was largely concerned to provide a list of such substances. The principal elements were gold and amber.

Paravinci-Bagliani (2000, 205) points out some important differences between Roger Bacon's writings on the *prolongation vitae* and the *De retardatione*, resulting in what he calls his 'extraordinarily audacious and coherent "theology of the body"'. For Bacon, humans can extend their span of life by drawing upon the empirical knowledge made possible by astronomy, alchemy and optics. In short, longevity does not have to depend on resurrection, but can take place in the here and now; the promise of prolongevity is natural, not supernatural. The experimental sciences, which Bacon defended and promoted, can repair the defects of human nature that resulted from their expulsion from Paradise with the Fall. Empirical knowledge would assist humans to manage their humoural decay, thereby arresting the apparently inexorable decay and corruption of the mortal body. In this respect Bacon's thought was revolutionary. It proposed that through science – in this case alchemy – men could gain control over their own natures and did not need to succumb to mortality, but these thoughts were indeed so radical that the proper understanding of the secrets of life should be reserved to those who have a duty 'to rule themselves and others'. These secrets should be entrusted to the few to rule over the many and, in particular, these secrets should be at the service of the body of the sovereign and the pope.

This prolongevist alchemy therefore played an important role in the evolution of Western attitudes. It involved a radical view because it assumed that man could achieve power over nature. Bacon's defence of experimental and empirical science against scholarly speculation was seen by his contemporaries as a revolutionary doctrine. Bacon asserted in his *Opus majus* that an 'extension of life' was possible with the aid of an 'experimental art' that could overcome the defects of existing medical knowledge.

## The Dietary Regime

Bacon's precocious empiricism and commitment to science against the fruitless speculation of idle clerics provoked great controversy, and he was eventually imprisoned in 1278 in Ancona, partly for his dissemination of Arabic alchemy. His work raised, in an acute form, the conflict between religious and secular views of the body. There is an important, albeit complex, relationship between the healthy body and the immortal soul. There is, apart from anything else, an etymological connection between the idea of saving the soul and the health or *salus* of the body. The verb 'to salve' means to heal a wound by an unguent or, in a more extended sense, to heal a person of either disease or sin. The theological notion of the verb 'to save' has a similar meaning – to deliver a soul from sin. The verb is related the idea of making something safe and we might be permitted, therefore, to draw a connection between 'to comfort' (i.e., to fortify), to make safe, and to salve. These interrelated notions therefore usefully bring out the connections between healing the body and healing the soul.

There is also a connection in Christology in the sense that Jesus is a prophet who exorcises devils, heals the sick and saves their souls. The idea of Jesus as a healer plays an important part in affirming the authenticity of the message of Jesus and hence, the New Testament account of his ministry is attentive to his healing powers (Davies 1995). It is perhaps unsurprising that Christians drew the conclusion that the healthy body was a sign of the healthy soul, and that deformity and disability were signs of human sinfulness. The etymology of the idea of malady is useful in pointing to both the presence of disease and the possibility of evil. Christ came to heal sinners, and it is ironic that there is in the New Testament the suggestion that Jesus may also have suffered from some debilitating

condition when he is admonished – 'heal thyself!' From these basic
assumptions, the view developed that there is a necessary
connection between the moral life and the healthy life and, in turn,
that people who conduct themselves properly (in terms of living a
'clean life') may expect to both live longer and to enter into heaven
having avoided such obvious sins as gluttony and lust.

There is, however, a basic theological problem here. If heaven is
the desired goal of the Christian soul, why not commit suicide in the
anticipation of accelerating entry into paradise? This was in fact an
option for Christians in the early Roman Church until it was
declared to be a heresy. There is, however, a second version of this
problem. It was notoriously the case that Popes had very short lives
and, hence, there was a recognized tradition that Popes were only
in office for relatively short periods. The solution to this puzzle was
to claim that the spirituality of the Pope was so intense that his body
could not house such charismatic power and that the inclination of
the papal soul was to abandon its mortal frame.

In later 'rationalized' forms of Protestant spirituality, however,
there developed the doctrine that the Christian soul had a duty of
care towards the body. There was, therefore, an idea of stewardship
towards the body. We can see this clearly in the pastoral advice of
Protestant leaders such as John Wesley. In Greek medicine,
diet (*diaita*, or 'mode of living') referred to the general conduct
and organization of life, including forms of dress, behaviour and
attitudes. In its more restricted sense of a mode of eating, diet was an
essential element of the Greek medical *regimen*. A medical regimen
is a set of rules or guidelines imposed upon a client to secure his or
her well-being. When the body is conceived as an input–output
system, the regimen restores the equilibrium of the body through a
regimen of purges, fasting, sweating and diet. Regimen also, of
course, has the somewhat antiquated meaning of 'government' and
is the root of 'regime', and 'regiment'. The *diaita* was a mode of living
set within a particular government of the body by medical practices.
Medical regimens imply an element of choice and responsibility on
the part of patients, but if we take a wider view of the whole process
of nourishment of the body, we need a more complex model. In
*Regulating Bodies* (Turner 1992) I developed the idea of a government
of the body from the notion of diet. In medical terminology, a diet is
a regimen of the lifestyle of the patient to restore health through a
combination of diet, exercise, moderation and relaxation. 'Diet' is

also, in political terminology, a government of the state. It was relatively obvious, therefore, to combine the idea of a diet of the body and a government of the state. A similar idea is to be found in Michel Foucault's theory of governmentality.

Governmentality had three aspects (Foucault 2000). Firstly, public institutions, procedures, calculations, and tactics permit the exercise of this specific form of power. Human population is its target, political economy is its principal form of knowledge and apparatuses of security are its essential technical means. Secondly, there is the formation of a series of specific government apparatuses, and the development of a whole complex of *savoirs*. Finally, there were a number of historical processes by which the medieval state of justice, converted into the administrative state during the fifteenth and sixteenth centuries, gradually emerged as modern governmentality.

Two important figures in the history of dietetics as contributions to longevity were Leonard Lessius (1554–1623), the author of the *Hygiasticon or the Right Course of Preserving Life and Health unto Extreme Old Age,* and Luigi Cornaro (1475–1566), the author of *Trattato della vita sobria* (1558), which was translated by George Herbert in 1634 and republished in 1776. Diseases are frequently interpreted as manifestations of a deeper malaise in the social structure. Just as cancer is often regarded as a disease of civilization, so obesity in the sixteenth and seventeenth centuries was regarded as a physical manifestation of the flabbiness of the social system, especially as it impinged upon the lifestyle of the rich. The disorders to which Cornaro drew attention were the 'bad customs' of the time, namely 'the first, flattery and ceremoniousness; the second, Lutheranism, which some have most preposterously embraced; the third, intemperance' (Cornaro 2005, 14). Cornaro, who was an Italian nobleman from Venice, saw the corruption of Italian cultured society by the Reformation, the falsity of court life and indulgence as leading necessarily to the corruption of the body. The solution to social and physiological pathology was to be sought in the government of the body through diet and discipline. Dieting, especially among the rich, was the main guarantee of health, mental stability and reason. A life founded on temperance and sobriety was the principal defence against the aristocratic affliction of melancholy and the disruptive effects of passion on reason. For Cornaro, therefore, the discipline of diet was formulated within a religious framework as the antidote to the temptations of the flesh. Cornaro and Lessius came to have a long-term significance for the development of a medico-religious discourse concerning the physical, personal and social benefits of dietary management.

The combination of leisure and luxury had especially damaging consequences for unmarried women in the gentry and, while serving women rarely suffered from melancholy, noble women were the principal victims of the English malady. Virginity and nobility both led to idleness and isolation, and hence to melancholy. The cure for this condition was marriage, diet, exercise and religion. When these failed to produce the remedy for unruly desires, physicians such as Robert Burton the author of *The Anatomy of Melancholy* recommended `labour and exercise, strict diet, rigour and threats' (Burton 1927, 273). The government of female bodies was thus linked via patriarchy with the government of the household. Since Burton (1927, 63) saw a great affinity 'betwixt a political and economical body', his dietary was necessarily a political treatise. Society presupposed a hierarchy of political control, descending from the state, through the patriarchal household, to the body and desires.

Many of Burton's anxieties and solutions were reproduced in the following century in the dietetics of George Cheyne, who observed that the expansion of trade and the growth of mercantile wealth brought exotic and rich foods into the market place. The result of these civilized luxuries was to 'provoke the Appetites, Senses and Passions in the most exquisite and volumptuous Appetite' (Cheyne 1733, 49). Cheyne's medical discourses were primarily addressed to the urban idle rich, who were the most exposed to the moral danger of strong drinks and exotic foods. The sedentarized life of the inhabitants of London and Bath provided a sharp contrast with the natural vigour of primitive man: 'When Mankind was simple, plain, honest and frugal, there were few or no diseases. Temperence, Exercise, Hunting, Labour and Industry kept the Juices Sweet and the Solids brac'd' (Cheyne 1733, 174). In order to reduce the destructive impact of affluence on the digestive system, Cheyne recommended, especially for sedentarized merchants and professional men, a strict diet, regular evacuation, exercise on horseback and 'a Vomit that can work briskly' (Cheyne 1740, xlvii). Cheyne's dietary regimen was intended to subordinate the passions of the urban rich, which had become inflamed by excessive consumption of rich and exotic food and drink.

While Cheyne was heavily influenced by Cartesianism and the iatromathematics of the Leiden school of medicine, he regarded diet, exercise and regularity as moral activities that promoted the control of unruly passions. It is therefore not surprising that his views were highly congenial to the religious outlook of John Wesley and the early Methodists. Cheyne's dietary regulation was easily incorporated within the Methodist code of ascetic behaviour and Wesley embraced Cheyne's medico-morality as the basis of his own *Primitive Physick* of 1752. Wesley also recommended Cheyne's *Essay of Health and Long Life* to his mother in 1724, partly because it was 'chiefly directed to studious and sedentary persons'. It can thus be argued that the traditional norm of fasting as an ascetic practice within the monastery was gradually transformed by the Protestant dietaries of Burton, Cheyne and Wesley into a suitable exercise of regulation for the laity, and that the elitist dietetics of Burton eventually reached the working class via the popular views of Wesley and his Methodist chapels. In the American colony, Cotton Mather (1724/1972) also published his *The Angel of Bethesda* in 1724 in which, while recognizing God's sovereign power over life and divine punishment of sin, he supported adherence to rational medical methods of temperance and moderation. Disease and disability were the normal conditions of old age and a sign of human imperfection.

The spread of dietary management into the home was eventually combined with the broader movement of general hygiene for the working-class family under the auspices of the medical profession. It represented a rationalization and secularization of food, which ceased to be a stimulant of desire and became instead, under scientific dietetics, a condition of efficient labour. The vocabulary of passions, desires and humours was replaced by the discourse of calories and proteins. The dietary requirements of specific categories of people became increasingly detailed and rationalized. Whereas writers like Cheyne had used very general classifications – the idle, the gentry and the sedentary scholar – dietetics now came to analyse the specific requirements of prisoners, workers, pregnant women, the schoolchild and the athlete. Each illness had its specialized diet – pulmonary tuberculosis, diabetes, allergic diseases and rheumatism all required individualized dietary regimens. Diets became specific to persons individuated by age, class, sex and condition. With this process, the idea of diet as a control of the soul in the subordination of desire gradually disappeared.

## Calvinism and Ageing in America

The Puritan leaders who established the early colonies in what became the United States appear to have enjoyed exceptionally long lives. In seventeenth-century England, men married in their late twenties and died in their early fifties. Consequently, they left unmarried children and did not live to see their grandchildren (Laslett 1965). In New England, parent–grandchild relationships were fairly common. Their good health and longevity may have been related to the plentiful nutrition and clean air that they enjoyed in the colonies, but in their eyes, their longevity was an expression of their piety. The ideal of Christian maturity was based on the idea that spiritual growth was always possible and hence they saw life as a journey punctuated by conversion, maturity and salvation (Cole 1992). John Bunyan's *Pilgrim's Progress* was the quintessential expression of this Puritan ideal of life as a confrontation of the Christian soul with the City of Destruction and the Slough of Despond on the journey to ultimate salvation. It was a pattern of physical decline and spiritual growth. This journey was set very much within the social confines of a patriarchal order in which there was a definite hierarchy of older people over youth.

Colonial America does not appear to have been characterized by intergenerational conflict. In northern Europe in the eighteenth century, the shortage of arable land, the growing population and increasing longevity created conflicts between fathers and their sons when farms were not handed down in a reasonable amount of time. In New England, land was readily available and, as a result, conflicts between generations were less intense. The patriarchal household of colonial settlement remained the ideal, but this situation was eventually challenged by the growth of the market, individualism and the secular values of the Enlightenment. Old age was eventually subject to a secularization process in which ageing became a health problem that could be managed by modern science. However, the result is that we no longer share a common vocabulary of ageing, and therefore the question – can we live forever? – is answered within a technical discourse which provides no guidelines for how to live, let alone why we should live.

Life is no longer a journey but rather a series of events, the meaning of which is either absent or disputed. Today's notions of ageing contrast sharply with the Calvinist ideal of Nathaniel

Emmons, a Puritan divine from New England who died at the age of ninety-five in 1840. Emmons is a central figure in Thomas Cole's historical and cultural account of ageing in his *The Journey of Life* (1992). At the age of eighty-two, Emmons finally resigned from the ministry and gave up regular preaching. He became an object of some curiosity in his old age, and it was recognized that with his passing, the old doctrines of seventeenth-century Calvinism with its insistence on predestination and hence the necessity to search our souls constantly for some sign of salvation were also passing away to be replaced by the more humane and universal message of Arminianism that characterized the Methodist revival. Salvation was available to those who freely accepted Jesus as their Lord. Emmons, while recognizing that humans had some degree of freedom to exercise their will, nevertheless emphasized human frailty and the urgent need for each soul to prepare for death. God could snatch people from this world at any moment and at His pleasure, and therefore our preparation for death could not be delayed or neglected. Emmons recognized that in the Old Testament, it was recorded that the patriarchs lived for a thousand years, but with our fall from grace, our lives were normally confined to three score and ten. Given God's inscrutable powers, the hope for longevity was an encouragement to wickedness. Given the frailty of human life, religion is an indispensable support in old age when our infirmities multiply and the surest guide for the righteous is to live a life of continuous and vital piety.

Emmons's late Calvinist world was challenged by the demographic transition of the population in which Americans could actually expect to live longer, and hence the religious attitudes of piety and humility gave way to the desire to employ modern medicine to remove the disabilities and afflictions of old age. The notions of dependence and humility were inappropriate to an age that emphasized youthfulness, activity and self-reliance. The attitude of religious leaders also changed to give greater attention to the conversion of the young and less emphasis on respect for the elderly. Whereas the New England Calvinists had developed an integrated view of ageing involving both loss and redemption, their successors had what Cole calls a 'dualistic vision', recognizing decay and dependence on the one hand, and self-reliance, virtue and health on the other. In late Victorian America, religion and hygiene merged to embrace a perfectionist view of healthy living.

Between 1830 and 1870 preventive medicine, hygiene, dietary reform and physical education came together to promote the ideal of individual health and medical self-care. Evangelical perfectionism was wedded to hygienic perfectionism. The prolongation of life became an overriding objective of health reform and the public health movement. The quest for longevity was not simply a medical objective; it was a moral one. It was necessary to eradicate addiction to tobacco, alcohol and sexual indulgence. Even coffee and tea resulted in an overstimulated nervous system that needed correction.

Piety and abstinence from substances that stimulated the system held up the promise of longer life, but how long could human beings live? Religious reformers gave specific examples of individuals who lived long lives – rather like Taoists referring to the Immortals – rather than resorting to statistics. Methuselah had lived for 969 years, Thomas Parr for 152 years and Luigi Cornaro for 98 years. Medical opinion in the nineteenth century, on the basis of autopsies of centenarians, averred that reaching a hundred years would not be unusual if people followed a pious and moderate life style.

American attitudes towards ageing and death therefore reflected a conflict and occasionally a compromise between two sets of values – Calvinist views about salvation, and Enlightenment attitudes towards the application of reason to human affairs. While Cotton Mather and Nathaniel Emmons were classic figures in the evolution of Calvinism, Benjamin Franklin and Benjamin Rush advocated the importance of moderation on scientific grounds. In his *Sermons to Gentlemen upon Temperance and Exercise* in 1772 , Rush supported moderation rather than abstinence, and in his medical publications observed that genetic legacy and moderation were the two principal foundations of longevity.

We can conclude this section on 'ancient techniques' by saying that while the Abrahamic religions – Judaism, Christianity and Islam – shared many beliefs and rituals in common, there are some subtle issues of difference between them. All three religions shared a common view of the materiality of paradise and immortal life. All three have a common respect for the wholeness and completeness of the human body in death. In contemporary Israel, this theological commitment to the importance of the whole body is illustrated by the development of *Zaka*, or the *Haredi* disaster-victim identification team (Stadler 2006). The social isolation of the ultra-Orthodox Jewish communities in Israel has come under considerable criticism, and in response, the Haredi have taken on the gruesome task of collecting together the shattered bodies of victims of suicide attacks, washing the remains and transporting the corpses to the Israeli Institute of Forensic Science. While this service is a new development and one that often involves transgression such as working on the Sabbath and touching dead bodies, it also involves honouring the dead. We can also see such 'deathwork' as religious resistance to modernity and secularism by placing religious practices at the centre of public space. Nevertheless, given the centrality of the physical resurrection of Christ, Christianity is perhaps most committed to the continuity of the physical body into and beyond death. Judaism appears to be more concerned with life in this world and with maintaining a variety of prescriptions and proscriptions about proper diet and conduct. In this respect, the Islamic distinction between *haram* and *halal* also points to the development of material piety in this life. We will see that, in the West, the modern quest to prolong human life by the application of science may perhaps be the legacy of Christian materialism with respect to the all-important survival of the intact human body beyond this world. If so, such a legacy is deeply ironic.

## The Moderns

In modern societies, a variety of medical techniques have been developed recently that are directly or indirectly relevant to the prolongation of human life. The possibility of reversing damage to the body and brain has encouraged the development of cryonics as one controversial technique that has been developed in the United States. The notion of preserving people is, of course, very old. The Egyptians mummified their kings and Benjamin Franklin recommended pickling the dead. The preserved body of Jeremy Bentham sits publicly on display in the University of London as a testimony to utilitarian rationalism. Cryonics is a technique to freeze people shortly after death in anticipation of future scientific developments that might restore people successfully with the use of molecular nanotechnology. At present, around 120 dead people have been cryonically frozen and some thousand live patients have signed up for what we might call 'cryonic storage'. The advent of cryonics might give a new meaning to the notion of 'the journey of life', since its advocates like to refer to themselves as 'cryonauts'. Critics cast doubt on the scientific assumptions of cryonics, arguing that it is difficult to see how such bodily damage could be reversed since 'ice crystals effectively turn all cells in the body into mush' (Brown 2008, 242). One solution is to flush out as much water from the cadaver and replace it with a fluid that will not form crystals. However, there is also the philosophical problem, namely whether 'the same person' could be revived since cryonics will not store memories. Cryonauts would be revived with no knowledge of who they are or what their past was. However, we cannot predict or anticipate what new technologies might emerge to resolve these problems. For example, Eric Drexler in *Engines of Creation* (1986) proposed using nanotechnology to overcome the problem of the formation of ice crystals. Alternatively, with DNA technology it might be possible to extract a nucleus from the frozen body of a cryonaut, inject it into a human egg cell and insert it into a surrogate mother. The same problems arise, however, with cloning, since it is not the self but the gene that is cloned and therefore such techniques might result in genetic survival, but the surviving cryonaut would be, to all intents and purposes, a new person with no memory of a precryonic self.

Despite these scientific and philosophical problems, cryonics could become big business, and in the States two companies – Alcor in Scottsdale, Arizona and the Cryonics Institute in Clinton, Michigan – already exist to promote its use. Alcor has developed a container that can house four whole-body patients and six neuropatients (or the brains of Alcor customers) in liquid nitrogen at −196 °C. This receptacle, known as the 'bigfoot Dewar', is an insulated container that uses no electrical power. Liquid nitrogen is periodically added to the Dewar to compensate for low levels of evaporation. However, according to Bryan Appleyard (2007, 203) both Alcor and the Cryonics Institute have suffered setbacks; for example, when several bodies thawed out in 1979 through lack of funds. The technical difficulties facing the cryonics business are daunting. For example, the customers who are signed up for storage must be frozen quickly after death, to avoid prolonged damage, and conveyed to an appropriate freezer. Customers who have suffered considerable trauma and damage after a stroke or car accident may face massive and expensive reengineering in the future. Nevertheless, enthusiasts will argue that cryonics offers the only available procedure for long-term restoration and, therefore, there will be a consumer demand for the procedure. In 2001 Alcor adapted cryoprotectant to produce a more concentrated formula that was designed to achieve ice-free preservation or vitrifaction of the human brain, and in 2005 this procedure was applied to the first whole-body subject. From these earlier experiments and developments, Alcor is confident that these technical problems of adequate storage can be overcome.

These developments sit within a much broader growth of social movements, institutes and scientific foundations that exist to promote what we might loosely call the quest for prolongevity. These include the American Academy for Anti-aging Medicine, which promotes mainstream medicine to explore longevity; The Methuselah Foundation, which offers the Mprize to encourage research into longevity; The Buck Institute in Calfornia which supports research on ageing; and SENS, which I have discussed earlier as one of the key British developments. Alongside these scientific institutions, there are more controversial developments such as the Extropy Institute and the World Transhumanist Association that advocate the scientific development of humans to such a point that they become posthuman. And then there is the Singularity Institute in Silicon Valley, California that seeks to develop artificial intelligence as a pathway to immortality.

The modern quest for immortality looks, in many ways, remarkably like the secular ambition of previous ages to use science (or magic) to extend life by empirical experiment. The craze for dietary prevention of ageing in modern societies looks like a modern version of the aspirations of nineteenth-century health reformers. The idea that we could experiment with cloning to give us immortality might resemble the hope of Chinese physicians to extend the life of the emperor with mercury. Perhaps the main difference is that the modern Immortalists no longer sit at the feet of the emperor or the pope, but at the behest of ageing, middle-class Baby Boomers in Los Angeles, Tokyo and Sydney. The quest for individual immortality fits the ideology of the postwar generations whose world view does not easily recognize disability, infirmity or death. The application of science to longevity and its treatment as a consumer aspiration is wholly compatible with the lifestyle and culture of the Baby Boomer generation who are only now reaching retirement and who inevitably will resist social irrelevance and cultural marginalization. These social conditions have combined to produce a generation that is fundamentally optimistic, but also secular and this-worldly (Edmunds and Turner 2002). There is an obvious connection between such values and the attitudes that lie behind the social movement to promote immortality. Death is no longer acceptable and ageing should be treated as a disease that is susceptible to medical treatment; indeed, extending life is merely the extrapolation of current medical practice. For Dave Gobel, the founder of the Methuselah Foundation, coming back to life would be merely like rebooting a computer.

The Baby Boomers had the advantages of a consumer bubble that did not burst. Michael Kinsley (2008, 39) humorously observes in 'Mine is Longer than Yours' that they found 'something approaching genuine happiness in material possessions' and their reputation for shallowness, competitiveness and greed was perhaps perfectly captured by a popular bumper sticker in the United States in the 1980s which read 'He Who Dies with the Most Toys Wins.' The quest for longevity can be interpreted as simply the quest to hang onto those toys.

The connection between ageing Baby Boomers and the quest for immortality is well illustrated by the life and publications of Ray Kurzweil who, with Terry Grossman (Kurzweil and Grossman 2004) published *Fantastic Voyage: Live Long Enough to Live Forever*. They promote the idea of a three-stage route to immortality. First, use all existing medical research findings to promote longevity: exercise, healthy living, sound diet, vitamin supplements and regular medical check-ups. Second, once you have achieved maturity, employ biotechnologies including stem cell research and gene therapies. And third, after this process, science will have developed to allow you to have recourse to nanotechnological repair, i.e., to apply engineering to reverse any ageing damage to your body.

Kurzweil regards ageing as a calamity that can be avoided, but he laments the fact that while many Baby Boomers will live beyond the 'critical threshold' of this generation, many will remain indifferent to or oblivious of scientific knowledge capable of preventing ageing. Kurzweil is, of course, applying this program to himself, spending one day a week in a clinic having medical examinations and taking a large dose of supplements every day. Kurzweil's generation has an overriding ambition – to avoid oblivion. Because the Baby Boomers played such a large role, at least on the cultural stage of the twentieth century, they are unlikely to embrace the oblivion of old age which the twenty-first century promises to give them.

Another important figure in the science field is Eric Drexler whose attitudes and aspirations also correspond to the Baby Boomer culture. Born in Oakland, California in 1955, Drexler did his early research at MIT, participating in the NASA summer studies in 1975 and 1976 on space colonies. During the 1970s he began to develop ideas about applications of molecular nanotechnology. In his 1986 publication *Engines of Creation*, he proposed to construct a nanoscale 'assembler' that would be able to build a copy of itself by the use of an arm and a computer. This development could lead to the efficient mass production of nanomachines.. With Christine Petersen, he founded the Foresight Institute in 1986 to prepare for nanotechnology. In 2005 he joined Nanorex to participate in their projects to develop molecular software. Drexler's work has been criticised because currently there is no way to build an assembler. Furthermore, while Dexler and his colleagues have produced some designs for simple machines, the design tasks and difficulties remain formidable. Finally, there are no reliable procedures to distinguish between the failures and successes of possible applications of these designs.

Despite these criticisms, the potential applications of nanotechnology are huge. In medicine, Drexler proposes that the development of nanocomputers would give surgery, for example, much greater precision and speed. Such machines could also be employed to help the immune system more accurately identify and combat cancer cells. Nanohealth machines could be implanted to correct failures of the aging body. Finally Drexler's machines could, as I have noted, assist in the development of cryonics since the resuscitation of frozen bodies would require considerable corporeal reconstruction.

## Conclusion

The modern quest for longevity, unlike its ancient predecessors, has little or no connection with religion or morality. The issue is simply to achieve immortality, or as close as we might get to that, namely living forever, by whatever scientific means are available. Whereas the ancients coupled long life with piety, the moderns have dropped the discourse of virtue and piety, replacing it with a concern for vitamins, supplements, exercise and stress-free living. The recommendation to abhor tobacco and alcohol for the Puritan divines was aimed at avoiding damnation, not choked arteries and failing coronary pumps.

However, as I have argued in this book, we should try to distinguish between living and surviving. Cryonics and other technologies might promise survival, but they have nothing to say about living, and without an understanding of living, it is difficult to justify the quest for immortality. For the divines, longevity was primarily a sign of possible redemption, but can the quest to avoid oblivion be a justifiable goal? The choice of the word 'oblivion' may be indicative of Baby Boomer values, because it is, to my mind, associated with the idea of celebrity, and as Andy Warhol said, we can all achieve fame, albeit for a few minutes in a lifetime. The quest to avoid oblivion represents a certain democratization of celebrity – a condition to which we can all aspire. However, 'oblivion' has no real content, and certainly no moral content, unless we could justify 'celebrity' in terms of some virtue.

This issue brings us back to the difference between survival (and oblivion) and living (and moral purpose). In writing this chapter, I have drawn heavily on two popular works – *How to Live Forever or Die Trying* (Appleyard 2007) and *The Living End* (Brown 2008). Both authors come to the conclusion that the real issue is not whether technology or medical science can really deliver healthy longevity, but whether we can find any meaning in mere survival. Appleyard (2007, 121) concludes that the extension of life does not in itself give life meaning and '[t]he awkward truth is that only religion can do that.' Similarly Brown (2008, 205) recognizes that mere genetic survival cannot answer deep-seated cultural and religious questions about our self-identity, and furthermore that the sheer boredom of endless existence would pose a serious threat to the sanity of life's survivors. While I do not think that religion has some superior claim on human meaning, I do think that the question of living raises moral and religious issues that science cannot (and does not aim to) solve. To quote from Max Weber's 'Science as a Vocation' (1991, 144):

Whether life is worth living and when – this question is not asked by medicine. Natural science gives us an answer to the question of what we must do if we wish to master life technically. It leaves quite aside, or assumes for its purpose, whether we should and do wish to master life and whether it is ultimately makes sense to do so.

Weber was realistic enough, however, to also realize that his answer did not really satisfy the radical students of his day who were struggling to come to terms with industrialization, secularization and, more urgently, the ravages of mass warfare and Germany's military surrender in the First World War. The young Max Horkheimer, listening to Weber lecture on the Russian Revolution in 1919, was deeply disappointed by Weber's adherence to this value neutrality that separated values from scientific facts. Many students flocked to the aesthetic message of Stefan George and his disciplines, but Weber dismissed their enthusiasms as unequal to the times.

The question that is pertinent to this study of ageing is whether, in a period that is undeniably secular, we can find any purpose to life that might justify life extension, and secondly, whether we could find any principles to justify the expenditure of resources that are necessary if such life extension is to take place at all. The following three chapters seek to address these issues more directly.

# Chapter Four
## The Political Economy of Ageing

They were not only Opinionative, Peevish, Covetous, Morose, Vain, Talkative, but uncapable of Friendship, and dead to all Natural Affection, which never descended below their Grandchildren.

— Jonathan Swift, *Gulliver's Travels*

## Introduction: The Demographic Threat

Let us simply assume that by 2050 the average life expectancy in the developed world will have increased by another ten years to around 90 years of age. The life expectancy of Japanese women will by then be well over 90 years. As a result, there will also be a dramatic increase in centenarians. We might reasonably assume by then that modest improvements in geriatric medicine and in the public provision of healthcare will reduce the misery of old age. These modest assumptions appear to be more realistic than Aubrey de Grey's assertions about an indefinite extension of life and rejuvenation. But let us consider the social and economic implications of both modest but continuous increases in life expectancy on the one hand, and a dramatic increase in longevity on the de Grey predictions on the other. How will advanced industrial societies respond effectively to either scenario?

What is problematic about the current prolongevity debate is that its champions rarely discuss the political economy of ageing – who will pay for it, what will be the unintended consequences, and how would it change the balance of power between generations or indeed between nations. One reason for this absence of any serious attempt to understand the social consequences of living forever is that the ideological underpinnings of the Immortalist movement are entirely individualistic and consistent with the values of the Baby Boomer generation that celebrate youth. In the drab early postwar years of rationing and restrictions, the Baby Boomer generation brought a new zest for life and enjoyment, but it has turned out to be a movement entirely consistent with the consumer boom of the 1970s. Although the Immortalist case is often wrapped up in a moral argument about the unacceptable nature of death – how can we let 100,000 people die each year globally of old age? – the ethos of Immortalism is essentially private and personal. It is not specifically concerned with issues about justice, dependency or economic growth. For example, the prospect of significantly extending the expectation of life in the affluent societies of the northern hemisphere by the application of medical research on stem cells has clear Malthusian implications for the world as a whole. There is a close relationship between poverty and injustice and, therefore, we should take this Malthusian question seriously if we are to understand the relationship between human rights and poverty. Although it is at this stage merely sociological speculation, one can nevertheless assume that, if successful on a large scale, the life extension project would produce a range of major socio-economic and environmental problems. Increasing world inequality between the rejuvenated, immortalized North and the naturally ageing, senescent South would further inflame the resentment of deprived social groups against wealthy aged populations. As the AIDS/HIV epidemic takes a significant toll on life expectancy in many impoverished African societies, the differences in the demographic profile between the North and South could become extreme. Failed states in Zimbabwe and Myanmar will only add to the extremes of wealth and poverty between societies. Unfortunately, life extension in the North implies increasing environmental degradation, global warming and consequently, further depletion of natural resources. In addition to social class conflicts over limited resources, there may be intergenerational conflicts over social resources, including conflicts over jobs, retirement benefits and pensions. As we will see, while much sociological research on generational relations has rejected the idea that increasing life expectancy will lead to intergenerational conflict, the life extension project raises new issues about such generational equity not covered by the current discussion. Whereas Malthus and Condorcet realized that there was an important connection between organic perfection and the improvement of society, the modern Immortalist movement pays scant attention to the social conditions that would be necessary to sustain large cohorts of human beings enjoying a prolongation of life.

A recent study drawing on world mortality data provided by the United Nations has shown that inequalities in life expectancy have increased between the rich and poor areas of the world since the 1980s (Moser et al. 2005). In light of this state of affairs, such inequalities would be aggravated by the life extension project and would be morally and socially unjustifiable in the spirit of human rights. There is a paradox in scientific discourses of rejuvenation. On the one hand, there is a wish to prolong life and on the other, there is an indifference to the means to prevent premature death. Assuming a link between wealth and health, it is unjust to value some lives more than others, i.e., to value the addition of extra years to already long lives rather than adding extra years to those whose lives are relatively short as a result of poverty and social conflict. While the quality of life for children in many African societies is declining as a consequence of poverty, authoritarian governments, new wars and the AIDS epidemic, lives of the elderly in many northern-hemisphere societies are being extended. The prospect of further life extension will simply increase this global gap between the rich and the poor. Considerations about existing inequality should moderate arguments about the health rights of the elderly to live longer and healthier lives, regardless of the unintended consequences for other communities.

The right to optimize longevity must be understood through the politics of human rights. Drawing on the human rights perspective, it is plausible to assume that the right to a healthy life beyond the existing natural lifespan could one day be feasibly supported by universal governing institutions. For instance, Article 3 of the Universal Declaration of Human Rights (Everyone has the right to life, liberty and security of person) can be used to this end. Political economy, however, has demonstrated that defining human rights is a political act that does not always resolve social conflict, and can actually aggravate it (Ignatieff 2000). It is thus very unlikely that granting the right to an extended life would automatically be beneficial for the population as a whole. Because there is an issue of scarcity in all human societies, the application of rights claims in one area can cause harm in another. For example, claims for an extended life by elderly parents may not automatically be compatible with the entitlements of their middle-aged children. Any political decision to add extra years to life by mobilizing a human rights agenda (such as anti-ageist policies or by reallocating general health resources to healthcare benefits) would neglect the consequences of such a redistribution of resources, enhancing the precariousness and vulnerability of other social groups. We cannot easily assume that all human rights claims are necessarily mutually consistent, or that rights claims can operate outside a zero-sum context. If we assume that scarcity is a necessary condition of any economy, then there has to be some process of distribution, but these processes do not necessarily guarantee equal opportunities. If we could guarantee that everybody (short of some unexpected accident such as a car crash) would live 125 years, then we would have achieved equality of outcome, but only a utopian environment of plenty could ensure such a state of affairs. With scarcity, there must be a struggle for resources – even in the richest societies of the developed world (Turner and Rojek 2001). In democratic societies, the struggle takes place between political parties and it is moderated by law. In undemocratic societies where there is no rule of law and corruption is widespread, the struggle over resources is typically vicious and the weak, such as children and the elderly, normally go to the wall.

Many sociologists have conceptualized concerns for social justice in terms of human rights. Because the scarcity of resources is an inherent feature of human life, redistribution measures aiming to attain social solidarity are institutionalized in order to protect vulnerable populations. Social justice concerns become problematic when high levels of scarcity entail moral queuing principles that prioritize specific groups over others on the basis of an implicit social consensus. A queue is simply a method of distribution typically based on the idea of 'first come, first served'. By a 'moral queue' I mean a principle of distribution based upon a shared system of values. A 'Do not resuscitate' notice on an elderly patient is one example of a moral queue. However, moral standards regarding human life are constantly challenged by new technologies (Latour 2002) that affect the foundation of human rights. If death by old age is perceived as pathological, it is likely that older adults will compete with other age cohorts for access to scarce medical resources. If, instead, death in old age is considered to be normal, then premature deaths in underdeveloped countries would in turn be interpreted as a priority since they are incongruent with the current norms defining the 'natural' lifespan. Moral queuing is thus central to the tensions emerging around the life extension project, because it establishes a hierarchy between humans that determines medical care. The question is – upon what shared values, if any, is moral queuing organized within the project of Immortalist longevity?

The utopian promise of biotechnology has been the object of many sociological critiques. For instance, René Dubois (1959) has argued that technological innovations commonly have disastrous unanticipated consequences, many of which are characteristically unpredictable. Similar caution must be applied to optimistic discourses surrounding the life extension project. Apprehension over this scientific programme goes beyond any traditional Luddite suspicion, because the life extension project threatens traditional institutions and values without providing any obvious reform or replacement of such institutions. It also increases social inequalities and social conflict. Biomedical technology has potentially far greater consequences for the status of the human than has been previously recognized. Once perceived as a vulnerable and marginal group, the elderly may, through rejuvenation sciences, be destined to find themselves in intergenerational conflict with other social groups, especially with youth, who are a declining proportion of most ageing populations.

Rejuvenation sciences, however, will be difficult to regulate, because of the mixed outcomes they have for individuals and for societies. Legislative regulation to limit the scope of anti-ageing technology would not be easily enforced for political reasons. In an ageing society, political parties seeking election will not stand against technologies that promise long life. In addition, it would be rational for an ageing individual to embrace the opportunity to extend life, despite the technology's negative consequences for society as a whole. Stem cell research is a good example of this problem. It is rational for an individual to want to add extra years to his or her current lifespan, even if this means spending much time bedevilled by geriatric disease and discomfort, while waiting for future cures for contemporary morbidity. We could imagine a common situation where elderly individuals are living longer, but with mounting problems from their (as yet) incurable geriatric conditions such as Parkinsonism and Alzheimer's disease. They hang on with the hope that a cure might be found. As such, societies will be subject the phenomenon of 'decompressed morbidity' within people's lifespan, including its economic, social and personal effects.

The moral arguments against the life extension project are considerable, even though a significant enhancement of the lifespan is at present remote. If anti-ageing technology can in principle make it possible to live forever, technology will corrode existing ethical systems, because there will be little motivation to follow a government of the body as the basis of self-regulation. Traditional ethical and religious systems have required what Michel Foucault has called 'technologies of the self' and a government of the body to achieve social order and personal discipline, but these conventional relationships between the ethical life, the good society and the management of the body are being dissolved by medical sciences. Traditional ethics assumed that we have, in some sense, a stewardship over our own bodies and over the natural world that supports our lives. The life extension project does not necessarily presuppose any personal responsibility for conduct, apart from compliance with a medical regime. The uneasiness that many have with this project can be understood through the moral legacy of religions on current value systems. For religious institutions, which constantly participate in debates over values, the life extension project presents a serious challenge, because religious communities have presumed the possibility of salvation and the enjoyment of eternal life on the basis of being virtuous and without sin. Rejuvenation sciences promise not an eternal sacred life, but an eternal, or at least extended, secular life. The life expectancy of an individual is not, in this scientific paradigm, based on moral worth, but on personal wealth or on the outcome of a political debate about the allocation of sufficient resources to meet the research goals of the life extension project.

We can also assume, with the application of successful life extension projects, therefore, that the ageing of populations of this magnitude will have a significant impact on the viability of the state since the tax base will be seriously eroded because there will be an imbalance between the working population and retirees. Even if retirement is postponed or made more flexible, there is a serious issue about how the productive population will be replenished. Longevity for the privileged generation will limit the employment opportunities of the young and increase the possibility of tensions between the generations. The citizenship claims of the elderly will no longer match their contributions to the system, if we reasonably assume that a person living until 125 years may still want to retire at around 80 years. Apart from elderly academics and bishops, there is little evidence that many people currently wish to be in full-time employment beyond 65 years of age.

The economic solution to the problem of an ageing population for developed societies is to continue to import labour from the less-developed world. We can argue that this strategy will be based on the assumption that the fertility rate of most developed societies drops to around one or below, and hence, if the economy is to continue to grow, such states must import labour through official migration policies. There is, for example, a large army of Filipino domestic workers in Singapore and the Gulf States, providing services to families with elderly relatives. Mexican migrants, both legal and illegal, feed the labour market in the states of southwest America. North African and east European migration has been important in the labour markets of northern Europe. Japan has been in recent years increasingly dependent on Korean and Chinese migrant labour. By 2030 we might assume that between 25 per cent and 30 per cent of the citizens of advanced societies will be over 65 years, that fertility rates will be below one and that the working population will be largely composed of temporary and illegal workers, constituting a large and disgruntled 'underclass'. These conditions will make the successful governance of societies highly problematic.

There are other solutions that involve delaying entry into the labour market by providing universal access to higher education and abolishing the retirement age. Another solution is to shorten the working week in order to guarantee more opportunities for employment for all. Another Orwellian solution would be a form of social storage by sending the elderly to gated communities outside their homeland. This is already a strategy employed by Japan, for example, where many Japanese retirees are now in retirement compounds in Thailand and Malaysia, where golf courses and medical care at competitive prices offer inducements for an emerging industry of geriatric tourism. The major solution in many of the Anglo-Saxon economies – the United States, United Kingdom, Australia, Canada and New Zealand – has been an attempt to dismantle the postwar welfare capitalist system of social security.

## Citizenship and Welfare Capitalism

In traditional societies with high fertility and low life expectancy, the survival of human beings into old age was a relatively unusual occurrence. There was no significant problem of dependency. Societies were exposed to a variety of natural threats that often seriously depleted population. In Europe, the Black Death created a significant labour shortage, and famine and warfare were sufficient to retain a balance between arable land and population (Ziegler 1969). Old age and retirement are products of the demographic transition (from high to low fertility and increased life expectancy) and industrialization. Citizenship and social welfare are in part responses to a new situation – how to provide for the elderly unemployed where relatives and kinfolk could not be relied upon to provide adequate cover. The social rights of citizenship were then closely tied to compulsory retirement, and these are contributory rights, since citizens are expected to make investments through social security payments to provide themselves with a modicum of protection in old age. These schemes have never been entirely satisfactory – with the possible exception of some Scandinavian societies – because the contributions have not kept the elderly out of poverty or at least out of considerable economic hardship. There is clearly a need for a 'new welfare state' (Esping-Andersen 2002).

Despite the limitations of social security and citizenship, Ralf Dahrendorf (1959) argued that industrial societies had avoided the crisis of capitalism predicted by Karl Marx because there had been an 'institutionalization of class conflict' and that citizenship had ameliorated the antagonistic interests between social classes. The societies of western Europe were relatively successful in the postwar period because they were able to combine three important ingredients to sustain social solidarity and citizenship: the production of resources to sustain a welfare state, the safeguarding of national identities and the protection fundamental rights. Globalization has in many ways undermined these three conditions. After the Second World War, there was a period of economic rebuilding on the basis of Keynesian policies of public investment for full employment. As the economies of Europe have become global, states no longer exercise effective control over corporations, and hence the tax basis of welfare is often eroded. Corporations can simply shift their investments to benefit from labour markets that are dominated by low costs – hence the huge influx of investments into China. Competition from Asian societies has contributed to deindustrialization in the West and put pressure on companies to outsource their production. National identities have been challenged by migration, thereby creating complex multicultural societies. Large diasporic communities of migrant workers have become an important feature of most European cities. Finally, states have often retreated from the protection of rights in favour of security and bureaucratic surveillance, and the squeeze on profits has resulted in attempts to reduce the social benefits of the working class. The need for security has resulted in a slow drift towards authoritarianism and regulation. For some writers, Singapore may represent at least one illustration of the evolution of this postdemocratic trend. Danilo Zolo (2001, 412) argues that in Singapore 'political representation is more than ever a procedural pretence, since the power is irreversibly held by the bureaucratic and administrative apparatus. Independent oppositional parties do not exist and there is no public debate.'

Singapore is sociologically interesting because it represents an almost unique case study providing evidence for the perennial sociological question: how is society possible? Many sociologists, following the sociological theories of Talcott Parsons, have been inclined to argue that, in the last analysis, a society exists insofar as there are common values. Given Singapore's history of migration and multiculturalism, it is unlikely that Singapore is held together in any significant way by a shared culture. Certainly we could not seriously believe that it has a common religious culture, since Singaporean society is deeply fragmented around religious loyalties. On the other hand, we would certainly not want to propose that the island society is held together only by coercive measures. It is true that there is an ever-present police force and quasi-military force on the streets, public transport systems and airport, and there is a coercive use of the law courts to control opposition and resistance, but this situation is very far removed from the coercive experiences of eastern European communist societies or contemporary China.

One important element of Singaporean solidarity is neither cultural nor political, but economic. Perhaps the social glue of Singapore rests ultimately on its pension scheme. The Central Provident Fund (CPF) is a mechanism whereby every citizen has to contribute towards provision for old age and sickness. This fund can also help individuals to purchase a property or finance an extra educational qualification. The system is crucial to citizenship since it encourages individuals to be responsible for their futures. Both employees and employers are compelled to make contributions to the scheme and, while the CPF has its own board, it is definitely subordinate to government plans. The policy has greatly facilitated home ownership and almost 90 per cent of policyholders have raised mortgages through the scheme. One important aspect of CPF provisions is the availability of free medical care in retirement. Elsewhere in the modern world where there is a considerable fear of the so-called 'ratio of dependency', namely, the number of retired persons in relation to those of employable age, the implicit social contract in pension-welfare arrangements has been challenged by the prospect of privatization. By contrast, the CPF is an economic and social contract that locks the worker into Singaporean society by securing their future well-being in return for their contributions. If pensions are collective arrangements that underpin social solidarity, then the CPF is a powerful mechanism for ensuring that individuals, regardless of race or religion, have a shared investment in the continuity of Singapore as a society. Singapore is of interest to political sociologists because it represents an interesting model of authoritarian, but largely successful, management and as such is taken has the harbinger of the future demise of liberal democracy as the model of successful development.

Pensions and social security schemes are important components of social solidarity in industrial societies that otherwise would typically experience higher levels of industrial unrest, civil disturbance and class conflict. Universal social welfare benefits provide citizens with a sense of membership in society and a responsibility for is continuing well-being. Pensions imply a social contract between the individual and society. Starting with the governments of Mrs Thatcher, the decline of union membership, the deindustrialization of the economy and the privatization of many public utilities such as transport, gas and water are economic and social changes that have brought the social contract into question. With the growth of a global economy, one general response to what is seen as a crisis of dependency resulting from ageing populations, declining profitability because of heavy taxation for welfare benefits, and declining productivity because of rigidities in labour law, has been to attack existing pension rights, mainly by attempting to encourage individuals to invest in private retirement schemes and to weaken the state's involvement in universal social security.

## The Neo-Liberal Critique of Public Pension Funds

In 1994 the World Bank published *Averting the Old Age Crisis*. It had been commissioned by Lawrence Summers, who had become convinced that it was necessary to question the public provision of pensions and to promote pension privatization along the lines of Milton Friedman's liberal economic agenda. One assumption of the report was that 'pay-as-you-go schemes' were economically unsustainable in the long term, partly because the payments of workers into the scheme were no longer sufficient to sustain pension benefits after retirement. The other defects were that National Insurance contributions deterred employers from taking on new workers. These problems were compounded by the decline in labour participation for people over fifty years of age and the obvious solutions, namely, to increase taxation and increase the retirement age, were unacceptable to governments faced by regular elections. In the West, it was assumed that the dependency ratio had become unusually adverse and that benefits were too generous. The report therefore proposed a three-pillar approach that involved retaining aspects of the mandatory pension scheme, a mandatory privately managed component, and voluntary personal savings.

While the economic thinking behind the report was that although workers would not accept increased taxes, they would make mandatory payments to occupational funds of their own choosing. Such payments are subjectively less negative than a direct payroll tax. Interestingly enough, while these changes to pensions were not forcefully resisted in the United Kingdom, they were met with considerable hostility in continental Europe. To some extent this situation brings out the differences between Anglo-Saxon capitalism and 'Rhineland capitalism' (Blackburn 2002). In France, Italy and Germany, there was effective opposition to pension privatization schemes through strikes and demonstrations. There were also a number of electoral defeats for right-wing governments that wanted to force through this style of pension reform. Among the working class, there was a strong sense that past contributions had earned them the collective entitlement to future benefits and there was also a clear sense of civic responsibility surrounding the defence of existing schemes. The social security schemes that had been in existence for a long time in many European societies were regarded, not as part of the state apparatus, but as part of a collective insurance plan.

The situation in the United Kingdom was noticeably more passive than on the continent and under both Conservative and Labour governments, pension provisions have been curtailed and reform has gone in the direction of privatization. British pension provisions date from the National Insurance Act of 1946. They have never been generous, because they are means tested. The United Kingdom has since 1945 suffered from low productivity, weak investment in manufacturing and an ageing population with a projection that by 2040 around 30 per cent of the population will be over sixty-five. Because, as a result, a large slice of public expenditure goes on pensions, Mrs Thatcher's Conservative government, which was elected in 1979, grasped the opportunity to reform pension provisions by pegging pension increases to prices rather than to earnings. The effect of this change was, in the succeeding seventeen years, to reduce pensions from 20 per cent of average male earnings to less than 14 per cent. This change, over time, brought the United Kingdom to the bottom of most league tables on public expenditure on pensions and it is projected that by 2040 British pensions will be only 5 per cent of GDP, whereas in some Scandinavian countries the figure is over 20 per cent.

Why was the Thatcher government successful in reducing public liability for pension support? One answer is that the British system was a relatively recent development and was not entrenched in the public awareness; very few people fully understood the implications of the changes and there was no robust lobby group defending the public scheme. Older voters tended to vote Conservative, and given Mrs Thatcher's large majority in Parliament, there was little political opposition.

One criticism of Labour governments has been that they produce high-tax and high-spending regimes. In the run-up to the 1997 election, Tony Blair's New Labour agenda stressed financial prudence and hence, the incoming government proved to be reluctant to restore the 'earnings link' with pensions. In June 1997 Frank Field was appointed Minister of State in the Department of Social Security with a brief to rethink all features of welfare policy. He favoured a pre-fund pension with responsibility for running them given to public bodies. The provision of pensions was to be universal, obligatory and without means testing. The view was that public pensions are an important aspect of social inclusion – a view embraced in the original Beveridge plan for welfare. After a period of political infighting, Field's ideas were opposed and he resigned in 1998. With the departure of Field, New Labour's plans for pension reform accepted some degree of privatization. This programme was influenced by Anthony Giddens's (1999) publication, *The Third Way*, which promoted the idea of shared responsibilities between the individual, the market and government in provisions for retirement and old age.

In the Blair years, despite the circulation of various policy documents and new legislation, the opportunity to develop a reformed pension system that could deliver both personal security and national savings was missed and personal savings remained stationary at around 7 per cent, i.e., below the levels achieved in France and Germany. Despite the rhetoric of creating a 'stakeholder society', the failures of the Blair government to significantly improve pensions were illustrated in April 2000 when the state pension was raised by a miserable 75 pence a week. Why did New Labour fail to embrace a genuine reform of pensions? One explanation is that voters over the age of 65 years have consistently shown more support for Conservative over Labour governments. In the 2001 election that confirmed New Labour in power, 40 per cent of those over 65 voted for the Conservatives and 37 per cent for Labour. By contrast, New Labour achieved 47 per cent support from voters under 44 years of age. One might cynically assume that there was little pressing electoral advantage in undertaking a thoroughgoing reform of pensions.

In many postwar societies, the dependence of politics on advertising and public relations and the dominance of the party machine over individual parliamentarians meant that the ideological and policy gap between contending political parties evaporated, making it difficult to detect real differences between, for example, Conservative and Labour parties. The use of focus groups and public relations strategies has the effect of moving all party programmes towards the neutral centre, thereby increasing political apathy and low turnouts at elections. The failure of New Labour to reform pensions may only be a 'failure' from the perspective of traditional Labour policies and, by contrast, it signifies a convergence in policies between the outgoing Thatcher-Major Conservative years and the incoming Blair-Brown years. Both wings of British politics had in fact taken up the position, however implicitly, that there should be less state involvement in education, health and welfare provision. In the so-called third-way philosophy, individuals are encouraged, and to some extent compelled, to take responsibility for their own futures. While this philosophy is certainly attractive from a liberal point of view, it fails to take into account the high levels of unemployment, the decline in labour market participation among the elderly, the inadequate level of productivity in British industry and the meagre levels of investment in industrial capital. Robin Blackburn (2002, 331) reminds us of one simple truth – 'In the long run good pension provision requires a healthy economy.' In 2008 the credit crunch, the sharp downturn in house prices, the crisis in the finance industry, such as the Northern Rock debacle, and the steep slide in the value of the pound, suggest that, in an economic crisis, the principle of taking personal responsibility for one's future may be inadequate as a solid basis for protecting the elderly against the vagaries of illness, disability and impoverishment. In the United States the credit crunch exposed a similar political scenario in which convergence over policies between Republicans and Democrats was further evidence of the erosion of genuine political debate, thereby confirming the dominance of commercial media over the public sphere (Nederveen Pieterse 2008).

## Intergenerational Relations

We need to see the issue of pensions against the more general issues of social solidarity and social security. These questions point to the fact that we should look at pensions from the perspective of intergenerational exchanges and the question of generational equity (Kotlikoff 1992). It is well recognized that the welfare states of Europe have rested on an explicit social contract between generations. This contractual welfare state is based on intergenerational transfers of resources through taxation and social expenditure. In addition to this public or formal contract, there is an informal and domestic contract between generations within households. Generally speaking, the state works to reinforce and sustain the informal contractual arrangements within households. With aging, declining fertility and compulsory retirement in Western populations, there has been, as we have seen, increasing pressure to modify the generational contract. Critics of the existing arrangements have argued that the Baby Boomer, or 'welfare generation', has captured the welfare state and its resources, ensuring that social funding is directed away from the young to the elderly (Thomson 1996). The social construction of a 'demographic imperative' is based on the economic assumption that welfare is a 'public burden'. Lobby groups in the United States have campaigned against public expenditure for the elderly and promoted the idea of personal responsibility and obligation within the family. Fears about a social burden have also been associated with the idea that there is growing conflict between generations over the unequal distribution of resources.

Alan Walker (1996) and Chris Phillipson (1996) in the United Kingdom have claimed that the notion of a demographic threat is being used as an ideological platform for a more general neoliberal attack on the welfare state in favour of both private insurance and greater personal responsibility for our own futures. What Walker calls the ideology of 'familism' played an important role in the Thatcher government's emphasis on personal responsibility for our own families and their futures. As state support for welfare has been cut, there is a greater burden on family members to provide care, but in reality, it is difficult for family members to undertake responsibility for the elderly, because the family itself has been changing dramatically. With high levels of divorce, increasing longevity and greater geographical mobility, families are too fragmented and diverse to provide the traditional care that occurred between children and parents in the traditional family. As life expectancy increases, often families may contain two generations of pensioners who need support. Walker (1996, 35) concludes by noting that although 'age-group conflicts have the potential for greater prominence in the decades to come,' whether or not such conflicts will be significant depends on how the state functions to enhance or undermine the capacity of individuals to provide care and support for family members.

Within a broader framework, there has been considerable discussion of the nature of norms of reciprocity (Gouldner 1960) and their significance for 'age integration', i.e., intergenerational solidarity. It has been claimed that modern societies are less tightly organized around age boundaries and as a result there is more 'age heterogeneity' in public institutions such as universities and in the work place (Riley and Riley 2000). This view of the breakdown of age stratification along ascribed criteria creates greater opportunities for age integration. In these debates, however, it is important to treat generational relations among kin as distinct but not separate from generational relations within society more generally. While one might take an optimistic view of familial affection and reciprocity, can we anticipate a decisive conflict around generational interests and cultures in the public domain?

The debate about intergenerational reciprocity can be usefully divided into two broad camps (Williamson, McNamara and Howling 2003). There is the generational equity (GE) argument that each generation should take care of itself rather than relying on other generations or the state. Privatization of resources is one logical outcome of this position. The alternative is generational interdependence (GI), which emphasizes the diversity of emotional, cultural and economic exchanges between generations and, in criticizing the emphasis on economic exchange, GI draws attention to the social importance of reciprocity norms.

The GE framework arose, as we have noted earlier, in the 1980s as a response to the perception of a looming economic crisis attendant upon radical demographic changes. This framework was associated with a number of conservative institutions such as the Cato Institute and the Olin Foundation. It also had an advocacy wing characterized by AGE (Americans for Generational Equity).

Their argument was based on the findings of empirical research, which suggested that, while the economic status of the elderly had been improving, that of their children had been declining. This framework argued both that existing provisions were unfair and, more importantly, unaffordable (Marmor et al. 1999). Dependency ratios between workers and pensioners showed, it was claimed, that current welfare arrangements could not be sustained in the twenty-first century and immediate action was required to provide for these demographic changes. It was in this context that economists like Lester Thurow (1996) predicted that age wars would replace class wars as the elderly use their political influence through interest groups such as AARP (American Association of Retired Persons) to steer resources towards pensions and healthcare and away from educational investments for younger generations. As age conflict increases, the possibilities for age integration decline.

The GI framework arose essentially as a critique of these pessimistic predictions about generational conflict. The GI position notes that the elderly do not function as an integrated and coherent category, but are divided, like the rest of the population, by class, gender and ethnicity. The interests of rich and poor elderly do not necessarily coincide. Furthermore there is little evidence that they vote as a block, and the interests of different age groups often coincide. For example, in the early 1980s young and old opposed cuts to education and health programmes (Minkler 1991). A recent analysis of data from the British Retirement Plans Survey undertaken by the Office for National Statistics on behalf of the Department of Social Security found that parents who help their children are more likely to receive support, that children respond to parents in need and that divorced fathers are the least likely to be involved in exchanges with children (Grundy 2005). Finally, it is unrealistic to expect each generation to be responsible for itself, because this ignores historical contingency. The generation of the Depression faced unusually hard circumstances that shaped its entire future (Elder 1974). Similarly, we may speculate that the current credit crisis and the turmoil in the American housing market will have a significant impact on young families who are struggling with a global financial meltdown which is not of their making. Research on generations clearly demonstrates that historical contingency means that we cannot assume a level playing field between generations and hence, the idea of fairness is not easily applied in these circumstances. The problem with the GE perspective is that it makes little allowance for vulnerable groups that do not have the resources to cope with exceptional circumstances such as natural disasters, economic recession or civil conflict. In all of these responses to ageing populations and resources, it is very difficult to see how social justice between generations could be achieved. Any significant prolongation of life along the Immortalist paradigm will certainly intensify conflicts over resources, even where these public conflicts may be absent within the family and the domestic household. Despite the cogency of the GI criticism, it is nevertheless the case that the GE lobby has been successful, because the simple logic of its appeal to individualism resonates with the neoliberal climate that was sustained after the departure of political leaders like President Reagan and Prime Minister Thatcher. The appeal to responsibility and personal choice against mandatory measures remains a potent aspect of the view that generational interests are on a collision course.

While sociologists and gerontologists have generally supported the view that intergenerational reciprocity, even with the decline of traditional family structures, is a significant aspect of modern societies, tensions over resources will inevitably persist, mainly because there is the suspicion that older, retired generations are parasitic on younger, employed generations. This dependency was humoursly portrayed by Anthony Trollope in his *The Fixed Period* (1882). In the novel, all citizens who reach the age of 67 years (the Fixed Period) would be deposited in an honorary college known as Necropolis, where they would spend a year of comfort, relaxation and reflection. After this period, they would be chloroformed and cremated, thereby avoiding the degradation and discomforts of old age. While Trollope's viewpoint was satirically presented in fiction, in real life the idea that the elderly are a severe burden and that solutions are necessary has had many takers. William Osler, in his address to Johns Hopkins University Medical School in 1905, praised Trollope, arguing that men above 40 years were useless and that universities should have adequate pension schemes to retire academics once their early creative period was over (Gruman 1979). The controversy that followed illustrated the underlying assumption that in a technological civilization, the economic contributions of the elderly are likely to be negligible, and in that sense they are a burden. The debate also pointed to the fact that by the end of the nineteenth century the issues surrounding age were no longer encapsulated within a religious discourse and that good health had become tantamount to secular salvation (Cole 1992, 173).

## Conclusion: Pensions for Longevity?

This discussion of pensions and intergenerational exchanges shows that the aspiration to live forever is deeply problematic from the perspective of social justice. How could any individual or society provide for such an extension of life with either private or public pensions investments? The argument of the Immortalists has to be that we can construct old age in such a manner that individuals could work for many additional years beyond the current age of retirement and that their longevity could be enjoyed relatively free from the disabilities and infirmities that currently attend the ageing process. But such an aspiration also presupposes that late capitalism can generate sufficient jobs to keep both young and old in more or less permanent employment if they are to accumulate enough capital to see them through to immortality. Such a prospect of working forever in order to live forever may not be entirely attractive, given current assumptions about the balance between leisure and employment. Does the Immortalist paradise require us to work forever? The economic conditions that must be satisfied for a large number of immortal individuals in the northern hemisphere to fund their extended life project now begins to raise equally serious questions about the psychological, emotional and spiritual issues that congregate around such a Swiftian scenario. If we assume that a third-way philosophy would be relevant to a world in which death was indefinitely postponed, can individuals, without significant state support, fund their interminable futures? How would the individuals of a future Luggnagg cope with such demanding and challenging economic constraints?

# Chapter Five

## The Moral and Spiritual Character of Old Age

To-morrow, and to-morrow, and to-morrow,
Creeps in this petty pace from day to day
To the last syllable of recorded time,
And all our yesterdays have lighted fools
The way to dusty death. Out, out, brief candle!
Life's but a walking shadow, a poor player
That struts and frets his hour upon the stage
And then is heard no more: it is a tale
Told by an idiot, full of sound and fury,
Signifying nothing.

— Shakespeare, *Macbeth*, 5:5

### Introduction: The Reward-Punishment Model

In traditional societies (by which I mean preindustrial societies in which religious notions were still authoritative, dominant cultural forms and where customary behaviour or 'morals' contained a strong component of psychological and social threat), good conduct on this earth was to be rewarded either by some form of life after death or by a beneficial release from the suffering of this world. By contrast, transgression of customary norms was threatened by eternal punishment, damnation or a miserable and indeterminate existence as a ghost or, literally, as a lost soul. There was a strong element of resentment in these conformity–reward moral systems in which the rich, who were seen to be proud and haughty, would suffer extreme miseries cheered on by the erstwhile poor. This spiritual resentment was expressed in the biblical maxim that it is more difficult for a rich man to enter heaven than for a camel to pass through the eye of a needle. As we will see, both Friedrich Nietzsche and Max Weber, in their analyses of religion, made much of this theme of resentment in the Judeo–Christian tradition, in which the weak achieved their final triumph over the rich and the proud.

The Christian religion added an important dimension to this religio-moral system by developing the theological belief that life after death would be corporeal in some sense. The Book of Common Prayer recognized the resurrection of the dead and the life of the world to come as essential components of Christian faith. The Christian hope is (or at least was) for resurrection in real, not metaphorical, terms. Christ came to save us from our sins in order that we would have eternal life, not as a transparent or lonely ghost, but as an embodied and justified person. The affirmation at the opening of the Eucharist – 'This is my body' – points to the centrality of corporeality to Christian faith. There are many aspects of this doctrine, but philosophically it rests on the argument that the continuity of a specific soul has to be conscious. It must also be in some way a continuous existence and it has to have a recognizable identity. The unique embodiment of individuals satisfies these criteria if, and only if, the person in the next world has a substantial resurrected body. The disciples in the biblical account demanded physical evidence of the existence of the resurrected Christ to restore their faith. Without Christ's corporeal resurrection, the promise of the Christian message was seriously compromised. In fact, it would have been exposed as a fake promise. There were many problems with the doctrine of the physical resurrection of the body, and medieval theology debated such questions as: Was the foreskin of the circumcised also resurrected when the righteous man arises from the grave? Could men that had been consumed by dragons enjoy resurrection? The destruction of the body of criminals, for example, in the opening pages of Michel Foucault's (1977) *Discipline and Punish* testifies to the premodern belief that this form of punishment not only killed the criminal, but prevented his ultimate entry into the next world. The criminals in Foucault's account of regicide had, so to speak, to be killed twice; they not only died horribly on the scaffold, but their bodies were so completely destroyed as to prevent any subsequent entry into the next world. Reassembling the bodies of the dead was therefore an important and necessary precondition for life after death.

The reward–punishment model of moral conformity was directed initially at subordinate social groups – slaves, peasants or workers. It was essentially an ideological aspect of social control (Abercrombie, Hill and Turner 1980). As we have seen in Chapter Three of this study, members of the dominant social classes often experimented with medical practices (elixirs of life) to gain immortal life. In the Christian West, the notion was that the human race had declined from the biblical paradise and, as a result, was confronted by the limited expectancy of life. The elites believed they could escape such a fate by the discovery of elixirs, but they also recognized that such medical interventions were in some sense the black arts – they were dangerous and these secrets should not be shared with the generality of men. The desire to continue life appears to be a basic aspect of human life – not overly subject to cultural, historical or contextual differences. Perhaps the desire for a tangible life after death was intensified in societies where life expectancy was low, infant mortality rates high and the infirmities of old age, unavoidable. The expectation of life at birth in England in 1561 was under 28 years of age and only 7 per cent of the population was over 60 years of age. Such conditions were probably conducive to aspirations for a better life to come.

In modern societies (by which I mean postindustrial societies in which religious beliefs have declining authority and where they have to compete with a secular scientific culture, specifically with medical doctrines about the nature of life), contemporary medical advances raise fundamental theological questions about the meaning of life and death. If we could in fact live forever, what is the theological implication of such a possibility for traditional notions about heaven and hell? In this chapter, I am mainly concerned with the moral, psychological and theological implications of the proposition that humans could live for indefinitely long periods, i.e., enjoy the benefits of prolongevity. My argument is that there is, in one sense, little change from the past. Life extension will be enjoyed by the rich, not the poor; by the powerful, not the powerless; by the North and not the South. One doubts that technical improvements in cryonics will produce cheap means of storing the dead or that a regime of vitamin supplements will be affordable by the poor in most developing societies. Prolongevity, if it is achieved at all, will also prolong the social divisions of this world.

In terms of morality and theology, however, the promise of longer life on this earth breaks the connection between moral behaviour and life expectancy. We do not need to lead morally upstanding lives in order to have a reasonable expectation of continuity. We do not need to be virtuous to enjoy longevity. However, good healthy practices, as recommended by secular science, may improve our chances. These lifestyle norms (jogging, not smoking, moderate consumption of alcohol, safe sex, and so forth) enhance longevity, and in this sense morality has been rationalized and medicalized. Sin no longer blocks the roads to eternal life, but obesity does threaten our longevity. But what about the more fantastic claims of utopian gerontology towards 'living forever'? In the conclusion of this chapter, I want to explore at least one possible aspect of prolongevity, namely, the prospect of spiritual boredom and the need to create a new morality, namely, a senescent ethic.

Much of this discussion draws heavily on the philosophy of Friedrich Nietzsche. The idea that the promise of heaven was in fact a feature of resentment by the poor against the rich has been taken from Nietzsche's doctrine of *ressentiment*, but Nietzsche's philosophy is ultimately optimistic, for example, in his notion of the 'eternal return' (the notion of *amor fati* in his *Ecce Homo*). People can enjoy self-overcoming only when they can embrace their fate without demanding it have any additional meaning. In *Thus Spake Zarathustra* (1969, 161–2) Nietzsche proclaims 'To redeem the past and to transform every "it was" into an "I wanted it thus!" – that alone do I call redemption!' In other words, life does not serve any other purpose. The experiences of living are not metaphorical steppingstones to a preferred future state of affairs. 'Living, like loving, must be its own reward' (Thiele 1990, 201). Something like Nietzsche's affirmative philosophy of healthy living in which conventional (Christian) morality is a type of disease might be necessary to give some life-affirming quality to mere prolongevity. However, the Nietzschean life affirmation for a life *Beyond Good and Evil* (Nietzsche 1972) will also have to address a theology of boredom. How will the elite who live forever cope with the endless repetition of the same without chronic ennui? Is there a medical cure for endless chronic mental fatigue? Can boredom itself become a spiritual condition? While utopian gerontology has been enthusiastically celebrating the prospects of living forever, it has yet to address fully these moral and psychological problems of fatigue, ennui, boredom and despair. Although I have sought to address these questions sociologically in the discussion, for example, of intergenerational justice, I return constantly to a theological framework, precisely because any discussion of interminable boredom has the same quality as any discussion of evil. It appears to demand an answer that goes well beyond the self-imposed limitations of a secular theory of existence.

## Body and Soul

In traditional societies, death, especially the ubiquitous but unpredictable presence of death in everyday life, was an essential feature of mundane expectations and religious practice. With rampant infectious disease, infantile mortality rates were high and life expectancy at birth was low. In much of northern Europe, the completed fertility of cohorts of women who were born at the start of the nineteenth century was five. The consequence was that women spent most of their lives coping with pregnancy, lactation and rearing their children. In Spain, for example, around one fifth of children born in 1900 died in their first year. With relatively short life expectancy, few children would have grown up to see their grandparents. In demographic terms, the efficiency of reproduction was very low. There is an anthropological argument that in societies with chronically high infant mortality rates, emotional attachment to children was not highly developed, because parents had to learn the art of 'death without weeping' (Scheper-Hughes 1992). While Scheper-Hughes's argument has been contested by anthropologists, it makes sense to assume that mothers in such circumstances would become emotionally indifferent to death which is a persistent and visible aspect of everyday life. Death, especially rampant and malevolent death, was an inescapable feature of the public domain, and this traditional world of dying is often contrasted with the more private, predictable and individualized form of death in modern society (Ariés 1974). Indeed, death is often hidden from view as the isolated elderly pass peacefully from life in the back wards of public hospitals.

In such traditional societies, the presence of death was a routine feature of everyday life and the promise of an afterlife had greater salience and immediacy. Death as an escape from the turbulence of this world was a significant feature of the medieval imaginary. This ever-present threat of death and the promise of life eternal were periodically underscored by plagues, famine and warfare; these were more or less constant features of medieval society. The Black Death created a new type of consciousness of death as an active agent, malevolently destroying human society. The centrality of tragic death in art and theology remained important ingredients of human culture. Reactions to the plague were obviously mixed, but they included a smouldering resentment from the peasantry that may have contributed to political unrest and anticlericalism in the late fourteenth century. Aware of the danger that society might collapse, the elite poured money into the Church as a key institution for the maintenance of medieval society. In more recent times, the prevalence of tuberculosis and the theme of early, tragic death sustained a consciousness of death in the literary imagination of the elite. Throughout the nineteenth century, the scourge of 'the white death' focused the minds of the cultural elite in Europe and beyond (Dormandy 1999). This aspect of western literary tradition in relation to early death found its romantic epitome in Joseph Severn's 1821 sketch of 'Keats on his deathbed'.

Given these difficult demographic and social conditions, millenarian and messianic movements were a common feature of traditional societies, promising a new kingdom to compensate for the deprivations of this world. In less dramatic terms, the Christian Church offered the promise of salvation and eternal life – under a range of soteriological doctrines and conditions. We know from the history of Western theology that justification can be narrow – the Calvinistic doctrine of a small company of the saved – or broad, in the Armenian doctrine of the salvation of all believers. However, the Christian doctrine of heaven and hell recognized a strong connection between moral behaviour in this life and the promise of salvation. The Ten Commandments were an essential feature of Christian ethical teaching in preparing men and women for death and eventual resurrection. In this discussion, I am, out of convenience, referring primarily to Christianity, but a similar theology of death and justification is shared more or less by Islam and Judaism. By contrast, the ancestral worship of many 'Eastern Religions' such as Shinto did not assume a corporeal resurrection on the Day of Judgement, and was more concerned to promote filial piety towards ghostly forebears. The concern of the living was to avoid 'hungry ghosts' and haunted households. The need to placate 'hungry ghosts' continues to be an integral part of popular Chinese religion, but it is clearly not compatible with Christian notions of 'the life of the world to come' (DeBernadi 2006). However, the 'world religions' in general developed an ethical discipline for mankind based on personal piety, the reward for which was the promise of some form of salvation, freedom from sin or release from the wheel of fortune. The Nicene Creed of the First Council of Nicaea in 325 and the First Council of Constantinople in 381 affirmed belief in 'the life of the world to come', which was regarded a central article of faith. Although the Nicene Creed has been rejected by many fundamentalist Protestant groups because it is not to be found in the Bible, it is evident that the doctrine of the resurrection and the promise of eternal life are building blocks of Christian belief.

There is no doubt therefore that the moral life of individuals was (at least in official teaching) regulated by the promise of heaven and the threat of damnation. This connection was often dramatically and compellingly underscored by artistic imagination. Perhaps the most important was the work of artists such as Hironymous Bosch (1450–1516) whose triptych of *The Garden of Earthly Delights* (after 1466) portrays hell as a bizarre surrealistic environment of hideous animals and demons. Although Protestantism abandoned such visual representations of hell, Baroque art and architecture of the Counter Reformation from around 1600 to 1760 continued with the visual contrast between the torments of hell and the leisurely, luxurious world of heaven. Such images of punishment and reward remained important in the Catholic world.

The doctrine of heaven served therefore as an official part of the Church's teaching on salvation, but it also played an important role in underpinning the Christian view of a moral life. Life in this world was primarily a preparation for the next; it was assumed that this mortal life was typically short and unhappy. Heaven was a reward for this-worldly asceticism and piety, but hell was also a punishment for the worldly and the wealthy. The Sermon on the Mount promised rewards for the lowly and downtrodden of this world, and greed or an excess attachment to material riches was one of the seven deadly sins, standing in opposition to the virtue of charity. Accusations of greed probably flourished in societies where the threat of starvation was never far away.

There is, therefore, another way in which one can read the promise of heaven, which was brought out in Nietzsche's theory of resentment in *On the Genealogy of Morals* (Nietzsche 1967; Schacht 1983). Because the sermons of Jesus declared that the poor are blessed, heaven can function as an aspect of psychological resentment. In a society characterized by grinding poverty and injustice, the resentment of the lowly is expressed through a millenarian doctrine in which the rich will be confined to everlasting punishment. It is the rich who have exploited the poor who will suffer, while the poor but righteous person will enter into heaven. Hell functions not only to reward good behaviour, but as part of a psychologically satisfying resentment against the dominant classes. A modern version of this argument might be detected in the robust pragmatism of William James (1922 162–3) in the *Varieties of Religious Experience* where he condemns the 'sick soul' for its 'manufacture of fears and preoccupation with every unwholesome kind of misery'. There is, he declared, 'something almost obscene about these children of wrath and cravers of a second birth'.

The promise of eternal life was a central feature of the Nicene Creed, and in societies with high mortality rates and short life expectancy, belief in an afterworld played a significant role in religious belief and practice. Christianity was itself originally a millenarian religious movement in which the expectation of a Second Coming and resurrection was a dominant religious theme of the early Church. The human body was a recurrent issue in medieval theological works including speculations about the physical survival of the Virgin Mary after death and about how devils possessed the human body. In Christian eschatology, there was a consensus that body and soul could not be separated without damage to human happiness and survival beyond life. As Aquinas also observed a complete person cannot exist until the body or matter has been restored to its while form at the end of time (Bynum, 1991, 228). Of course the doctrine of physical resurrection raised acute conceptual difficulties for Christian theologians. Would, for example, the fingernails of an individual all be restored with resurrection? Could a person eaten by a dragon enjoy physical resurrection? The issue of the resurrected body was not, of course, merely a speculative issue for theologians. It formed the basis of popular religious belief and practice with respect to the relics of saints, their miraculous healing of the laity. In these respects, Christianity has a decisively corporeal cosmology of the world.

## Body, Self and Society

The sociology of the body has generally attempted to show that the metaphors of good health also apply to social organization. An effective corporation is thus said to be lean and mean. There are, however, two more fundamental issues to consider. The first is the orthodox doctrine of the Christian Church involving a belief in the resurrection of the body. In modern theology after Rudolf Bultman's programme of the demythologizing of Christian belief, there is probably a tendency to treat 'resurrection of the body' as metaphorical statement about immortality, but in traditional theology the resurrection was understood to be a factual statement about the tangible existence of the body as a miracle of the resurrection. Otherwise, the resurrection of Christ cannot function as a fundamental confirmation of his divinity. If Christ only metaphorically emerged from the tomb, it is difficult to make sense of the faith that is so powerfully manifest in the Gospels. The continuity of a ghostly and immaterial soul is not part of the evangelical faith of the Christian gospel.

The Christian view of life after death raises complex issues about our personal identity, namely, that the doctrine of physical resurrection is the only guarantee of spiritual continuity. The Christian doctrine assumes not my general or indeterminate salvation, but something very particular, namely, that if I am to enter into eternal life, it is eternal existence of a specific person. If it is not this specific form of justification, why would I lead a moral life at all?

Religious or spiritual continuity requires some manifestation of the continuity of a specific, historical and unique being. I assume that the New Testament story of the resurrection of Jesus has this notion of specific identity. The narrative of Christ's reappearance in material form is told very graphically in the account of Thomas's doubt when he put his hands into the wounds of Christ. One cannot hope for a more corporeal account than that, but in order for the wounds to prove Christ's resurrection, Thomas must recognize Jesus the man by his shape, size and comportment. He has to recognize the embodied Jesus; otherwise how could we be sure that Thomas had not by mistake encountered a wounded person whom he mistakenly thought was Jesus? The doctrine of physical resurrection is necessary to overcome a problem of identity. My continuity after death requires (in some sense) my (more or less) continuous embodiment. The alternative position would entail some belief in a ghostly presence floating inconsistently between this world and the next. Belief in ghosts has never been an aspect of orthodox Christian doctrine, and following the work of the French philosopher Jean-Luc Nancy (2003, 27), we can say that Christianity is a religion of the tangible – 'Christianity will have been the invention of the religion of touch, of the sensible, of the immediate presence to the body and to the heart.'

The body, or more specifically, embodiment, cannot be divorced from the self, especially from the idea of the self existing over time. Who I am, from a sociological point of view, depends on other people routinely and unambiguously recognizing me in social encounters. Persistent misrecognition would lead to confusion, anger and eventually paranoia. It has become fashionable in sociology to 'deconstruct' the self, thereby denying its coherence or continuity. In terms of everyday practice, however, it is difficult to see how the fragmentation of the self could be a viable condition of successful interaction. One reason why misrecognition is not a persistent feature of everyday life is that I recognize people by the very facticity of their embodiment. The nexus between body, self and society is sufficiently tight to minimize misrecognition. This phenomenal fact of everyday life is also the condition under which I recognize myself as myself. If my body changed uncontrollably over short periods of time – rather like a human chameleon – I would not be able to recognize myself. The same sociological and phenomenological conditions apply to life after death at least in the

Christian framework of resurrection. I must be sufficiently embodied continuously to know that I have been resurrected and not become somebody else.

What is the implication of this philosophical discussion? There is, in traditional religious systems, an important connection between health, longevity, morality and sanctity. In the Christian doctrine of justification, the saints have mastered their bodies and their souls. Christian theology does not in fact create a gulf between moral behaviour, healthy living and life after death. In this respect, it did not recognize any hiatus between 'the good life' of the body in this world and resurrection in the next. There was, with respect to justification, a clear relationship between how we behave towards our bodies in this life and the expectation of life everlasting. This connection could be based either on moral self reflection – I shall get my just rewards for my conduct in this mortal life – or on resentment – the rich and powerful will be punished hereafter.

We can express this somewhat complex picture in terms of simple demography. In the majority of traditional societies, a long life was the exception. There was, therefore, a dramatic relationship between a short life in the secular here and now, bracketed by either oblivion or eternity. Of course, strict Calvinism said nobody can know whether they are in the Elect, and no 'good works' can guarantee immortal bliss. According to Weber's (1930) *The Protestant Ethic and the Spirit of Capitalism*, the bleak and brutal picture of Calvinism was modified to suggest that riches were indeed a sign of election. We could re-read the Weberian narrative to suggest that a healthy life based on ascetic restraint resulted in secular longevity and the hope of paradise. It is within this framework that I want to consider the implications of ageing and the possible arrest of ageing by life prolongevity.

The new biological technology goes to the core of Nietzsche's views on morality and the 'overman'. Can biology replace morality by allowing us to live forever, regardless of our behaviour in this world? If medicine can offer a certain cure for such conditions as venereal disease, lung cancer and obesity, would I change my behaviour towards my sexual partners; would I abandon my preference for cigars and chocolate cakes in favour of asceticism? Why not opt for a sexually active old age with multiple partners with the assistance of Viagra? The new medical technologies imply that human beings could in principle live forever and, therefore, if the new biological sciences make the idea of living forever a real possibility, then we can have a life beyond ethics. The Christian idea of an afterlife and the Buddhist quest for release from the cycle of rebirth would both become problematic obscure beliefs. For example, it is difficult to see how the ethical determinism of Buddhist doctrine could survive the genetic determinism of modern medical sciences. Technology thereby breaks the relationship between ethics and the bodily regulation of life. If we can live forever through medical technologies, why bother with ethics?

## The Theology of Boredom

The utopian aspect of scientific technology declined in the twentieth century as the prospects of nuclear disaster and environmental pollution became dominant aspects of public debate. This public unease with scientific advance has been reflected in opposition to genetically modified food and in growing awareness of the hitherto unforeseen consequences of global warming. This lack of confidence and trust in science possibly explains the academic success of the concept of 'risk society' as a general explanation of our dilemma (Beck 1992). In this discussion of technology and the body, I have tried to suggest that current stem cell research has potentially far greater consequences for society and the status of the human.

Such research is difficult to regulate because its medical results appear to promise untold benefits to the ageing individual. Stem cell research perfectly illustrates an interesting problem in the idea of rationality. It is rational for me as an individual to want to live forever, even if this means that I shall spend much of my life bedeviled by geriatric disease as I wait for future cures for my contemporary morbidity. One example would be the prevalence of Type 2 Diabetes in affluent societies, especially among the elderly. We could imagine a situation where stem cell research has cured various forms of heart disease, Parkinson's disease and high blood pressure, but it has found no cure for diabetes. We are living longer, but with mounting problems from our (as yet) incurable diabetes. This tension between increasing longevity and mounting morbidity takes us back to the Greek myth of Tithonus – can modern medicine not only keep me alive longer, but provide solutions that will allow me to remain young?

The prospects of living forever are at present remote, and the moral arguments against such a goal are considerable. It is here also that Martin Heidegger's notion of boredom in *The Fundamental Concepts of Metaphysics* (1995) might become useful. Prolonged life with no purpose will result in a profound boredom when we are trying to kill time or passing the time by diversions. Heidegger believed, however, that at the end of this process there was the possibility that one could find an emptiness that would release one from boredom. From Heidegger we might develop a more positive notion of ageing in terms of his third stage of boredom and we might no longer thereby make demands on social life but rather acquire a greater capacity to deal with ageing. This development is, with modern technology, an unlikely outcome. If medical technology can in principle make it possible, at least for the affluent West, to live forever, technology will corrode ethics, because there will be little motivation to follow an ethical diet, i.e., a government of the body. At least, religious culture will be undermined by the prospect of an eternal secular life, even if that secular existence is one of boredom and discomfort. At this point, humanity will have progressed well beyond the conventional division between culture and technology, and the division between animality and humanity will become meaningless.

One pessimistic conclusion would be that while the life span could be extended indefinitely, it would expose human beings to significant mental instability and infirmity. The boredom that would be associated with the endless repetition of life might be intolerable and as people become bored with life as well as bored from life, it is unlikely that psychiatric medicine could discover antidepressive drugs that could inoculate us against perpetual ennui. The other issues are moral, namely the sheer injustice of the current prospects of prolongevity where both the average lifespan and life expectancy of sub-Saharan Africa have declined significantly against northern hemisphere changes.

Can we assume that a new senescent ethics would be developed in response to these dystopian changes? Let us turn to Michael Raposa's (1999) *Boredom and the Religious Imagination*. Raposa identifies different levels of boredom: being bored by something or we can be bored by ourselves. In these circumstances, we are forced to 'spend time' or 'kill time'. It is here that one can see the overwhelming threat of prolongation – how much time can one kill? However, turning to Heidegger's (1995) *The Fundamental Concepts of Metaphysics*, Raposa identifies a deeper level of boredom, where the world becomes boring for one in which 'nothing matters'. In this deep boredom of the world, one can enter a spiritual state of indifference. This spiritual boredom can lead to transcendence and overcoming, when we are liberated from the particular character of the here and now. We are no longer caught up in trivial tedium, but in a more profound boredom that exposes the real nature of existence. But Heidegger's notion of a revelatory boredom means that we recognize ourselves as beings-toward-death. This notion of a spiritual boredom still requires, therefore, an end to life, which prolongevity seeks to deny.

The individualism and secularist naivety of the Immortalist position has been challenged by leading figures philosophy such as Bernard Williams (1973), who claimed in particular that indefinite longevity would lead to intense boredom with the self. Of course, the Immortalist movement has attempted to address this question of boredom, but characteristically from a practical–medical rather than theological–moral angle. There are several solutions to the boredom problem that have been considered. Alan Harrington (1973) suggests that we could have long periods of hibernation or prolonged sleep that could be programmed to overcome boredom. David Pearce (2005), the co-founder with Nick Bostrom of the World Transhumanist Association and founder of the Abolitionist Society, in an interview in *Nanoaging* offered several counterpositions to the issue of boredom. First, he believes that with the development of 'designer babies', we can, in principle, eliminate the genes that are associated with anxiety disorders, depression and general malaise. We can, in short, breed people who are better able to withstand the boredom that afflicted earlier generations. He also believes that the creative development of psychopharmacology can help us engineer drugs that would enable us to cope with the threat of a tedious existence. A better understanding of the emotions will also result in more sophisticated treatment of mood disorders. Finally, 'Prosperty's control of the neurochemistry of time perception should allow our descendants to live subjectively as long as they choose everyday of their lives. Posthumans won't apprehend time in the manner of their primate ancestors' (Pearce 2005, 3). Advances in chemistry, it is claimed, will allow us to solve the problems faced by Gulliver's immortal inhabitants of Luggnagg, and this indefinite extension of life can be achieved without any increase in human virtue. The ironic message of Swift's fable was that old age ought to be accompanied by an increase in wisdom and virtue, but the Immortals of Luggnagg had neither. Without some retraining or virtue, won't the Immortals of some future age merely revert to their old habits, becoming bored with living forever? Pearce certainly recognizes this issue as something that has to be solved. He ruminated on the fact that, for example, following the euphoria of winning the lottery, after a few weeks people simply revert to their old lifestyles as if nothing significant had happened. He admitted that '[l]ikewise, following a short-lived burst of euphoria at being granted eternal youth, something analogous might befall us too. As our emotional thermostats kicked in, we might be almost as malaise ridden as before. Unless we recalibrate the mind's hedonic tone, our quality of life as quasi-immortals won't be much higher than our quality of life as lived for three score years and ten' (Pearce 2005, 10). One problem with this type of medical optimism is that past attempts to develop a pharmacological solution to depression have been at the very least controversial and often disastrous. The history of lifestyle drugs such as Prosac and Paxil would be significant examples of such failures (Turner 2004).

## Conclusion: Generational Change and the Theology of Happiness

At the beginning of this chapter, I distinguished, admittedly in a rather crude manner, between two stages of religious evolution. In societies with short life expectancy and a short but miserable period of ageing, one would anticipate the growth of religions that compensate the tragedy of this world with the bright promise of life everlasting after death. Such religions typically have a theology of unhappiness. The old Calvinist view of the salvation of the elect would be the high-water mark of this type of theology. Our world is very different. There are three important social changes that have radically changed Britain and much of the developed world in the modern period: demographic, religious and economic. Since the late nineteenth century, in what Laslett (1995) called the 'secular shift from the 1880s to the 1980s', life expectancy for males in England and Wales climbed steadily from 44.2 to 71.0 years. Secondly, in this period there was also a remarkable secularization of Britain in the second half of the twentieth century in which attendance at church, daily prayer and belief in life after death declined significantly (Martin 1967; Wilson 1966). Thirdly, since the late 1970s consumerism intensified with financial liberalization, an emphasis on youth cultures and the aestheticization of everyday life (Featherstone 2007). Over the last century, belief in the inevitability of old age and the assumption that ageing meant declining physical and mental powers were questioned and criticized. In addition, compulsory early retirement largely disappeared from the advanced industrial societies to be replaced by doctrines of positive ageing, flexible retirement and increasing leisure. The new emphasis on prolongevity, if not immortality, can be seen as simply an extension and consolidation of this social and cultural revolution.

The new optimistic mood of medical progress is essentially a product of the fact that with the new century, the Baby Boomers are in their sixties and planning a new socio-biological future for themselves. The consumer society of the Baby Boomer generation requires a new theology which I have called a theology of happiness that celebrates their social and economic power and their reluctance to hand over to the next generation the benefits they have enjoyed since the 1950s. The Baby Boomers are essentially a secular generation; their progress through the second half of the twentieth century was accompanied by a decline of traditional, institutional forms of Christianity. The idea that all social and human problems can be fixed by the correct technology and planning is a secular assumption. 'Generation' is here defined as an age group whose common identity and experiences have been shaped either by traumatic events (such as trench warfare in the First World War) or by some major social changes (such as the effects of the Great Depression). The Baby Boomers can only be loosely defined in chronological terms, but I am assuming they are people born in the three decades after 1945, whose values and outlook were shaped profoundly by the consumer culture, the Bay of Pigs fiasco, the Kennedy assassination, the Vietnam War, the student revolts and the peace movement (Turner 2006b). They were also the first global generation in the sense that the experience of postwar reconstruction and consumerism came eventually to shape most of the societies of the developed world, including Japan (Edmunds and Turner 2005). The quest for spirituality and individual meaning appears to be more characteristic of the generation that came after the Baby Boomers. Perhaps the revival of religious piety and faith that we have witnessed in the last two decades is in part a reaction against the secularism and worldliness of the Baby Boomers. Since 9/11 we can also detect an obvious shift in global culture away from hedonism and cosmopolitanism towards a greater emphasis on security and nationalism, namely, to what I have called 'the enclave society' (Turner 2007). We can predict that a new generational culture may now begin to coalesce around these new issues – environmental degradation, conservation, international migration, national security and economic stability – and whose values will be clearly different from those of the Baby Boomers.

For these new generations, the attack on the Twin Towers, the war on terror and the credit crunch will be defining events that have in some measure closed off or curtailed opportunities and resources that the Baby Boomers took for granted. The notion that we can live forever is high on the personal and collective agenda of people in their sixties, who can probably better weather the storm of global economic downturn than younger age groups. The postwar generation is still living in a world where things – problems, puzzles and issues – can be fixed by secular means. In the Immortalist world, where ageing can be controlled by what we might call iatroengineering and the meaning of death has been fundamentally transformed, death will be increasingly the result of accident or suicide. Perhaps this may explain, in part, the extraordinary display of national grief in Britain following the death of Lady Diana Spencer. The People's Princess was in some respects representative of a new British youthful culture that was stylish, energetic, anti-establishment and cosmopolitan. She held out an alternative vision of what the Crown might symbolize in a postmodern, postcolonial Britain. Her death was seen as tragic, untimely and unnecessary. Its very accidental quality was consistent with the Immortalist doctrine that with proper medical planning, life can be fully planned and death wholly banished. A natural death is replaced by the tragic event of death by accident.

We can now see that the movement to achieve indefinite life is, in fact, perfectly compatible with medical ethics. Thus, for example, the two principles of beneficence (the doctor should be well-intentioned and aim to do good towards the patient) and nonmaleficence (the doctor must avoid harming the patient) are compatible with the idea that the doctor should take all measures necessary to keep the patient alive and in a comfortable condition. These ethical principles have also, of course, made it difficult for many medical professional associations to support legislation in support of euthanasia. The fundamental ethical principle in support of euthanasia is the idea that the doctor must respect the autonomy of the patient, thereby treating the patient as a rational being. The notion of patient autonomy is not absolute, since, if a doctor decides that a particular treatment is futile or harmful, he can deny the patient's access to the treatment. Within the law, the sanctity of life often triumphs over a patient's wish to die. The right to life tends to triumph over the right to die. The growth of palliative care will further stand in the way of the right of a conscious and rational patient to die rather than suffer from an incurable disease. Therefore, the assumption upon which the case for 'palliative care rather than physician-assisted death rests is that it is always better to live than to die, even if one passionately wants to die' (Warnock and Macdonald 2008, 14). The ethical culture of medicine will on the whole support research that extends life, especially if the 'incurable diseases' of the elderly can, in fact, be cured or controlled. Medical ethics in this respect can be employed by Immortalists to argue that the quest to save life is unquestionably a moral principle and, hence, longevity requires no further ethical justification. To save life is the supremely moral act. There is, however, one principle of the four fundamental principles of medicine that might challenge this scenario, namely, the principle of justice, in which a doctor must allocate scarce resources fairly between his or her patients. In the next chapter I turn to the issue of allocating healthcare on the basis of age.

# Chapter Six

## Vulnerability and the Ethic of Care

What does not kill me makes me stronger.

— Friedrich Nietzsche,
*Twilight of the Idols*, 23

### Introduction: Vulnerability, Precariousness and the Body

In thinking about the human condition, we must keep in mind four fundamental aspects of our existence that follow from our embodiment: the vulnerability of human beings as embodied creatures, the dependency of humans (especially during their early childhood development), the general reciprocity or interconnectedness of social life and finally, the precariousness of social institutions. There is a dialectical relationship between these four components that becomes obvious when one thinks about the process of technological modernization. Within this dialectical balance between vulnerability, dependency, reciprocity and precariousness, modern technologies, especially medical technology, have powerful, unpredictable and far-reaching implications, and they are largely disruptive of the relationship between the four components. If our embodiment is the real source of our common sociability, then changes to embodiment must have significant implications for both vulnerability and inter-connectedness. The new microbiological revolution in medical sciences holds out the promise of long life and rejuvenation, but the prospect of living forever is driven by a powerful commercial logic and has (largely unrecognized) military and security applications and implications that are problematic for human rights and democracy. New medical procedures such as therapeutic cloning, new reproductive technologies, rejuvenative medicine, stem cell research applications, cryonics, fetal surgery and organ transplants create the possibility of a medical utopia, but they also reinforce social divisions and inequalities, especially between rich and poor societies. This chapter raises two fundamental political questions: What are the proper ends of a political community, and does the current biotechnological revolution anticipate, following Michel Foucault (1970) in *The Order of Things*, the end of Man? Will 'man' be eventually 'erased, like a face drawn in sand at the edge of the sea' (Foucault 1970, 387)?

Human beings are vulnerable and insecure, and their natural environment, precarious. In order to protect themselves from the uncertainties of the everyday world, they must build social institutions (especially political, familial and cultural institutions) that come to constitute what we call 'society'. We need trust in order to build companionship and friendship to provide us with means of intimate mutual support. We need the creative force of ritual and the emotional ties of common festivals to renew social life and to build effective institutions, and we need the comforts and supports of social institutions as means of fortifying our individual existence. Because we are biologically vulnerable, we need to build political institutions to provide for our collective security. These institutions, however, are themselves precarious and cannot work without effective leadership, political prudence and good fortune to provide an enduring and reliable social environment. Rituals typically go wrong; social norms offer no firm or long-term blueprint for action; and the guardians of social values – priests, academics, lawyers and others – turn out to be open to corruption, mendacity and self-interest. However, the afflictions of everyday life also generate intersocietal patterns of dependency and connectedness, and in psychological terms, this shared world of risk and uncertainty results in some degree of sympathy, empathy and trust without which society would not be possible. All social life is characterized by this contradictory and delicate balance between scarcity, solidarity and security. This theory of society embraces a set of Hobbesian assumptions, in which life is vulnerable, i.e., nasty, brutish and short. It does not follow, however, that we are forced to accept the individualistic assumptions of a Hobbesian social contract. Instead, human and social rights are juridical expressions of social solidarity, whose foundations are in the common experience of vulnerability and precariousness.

Following Pierre Bourdieu (2000) in his *Pascalian Meditations*, we acquire practical reason through the everyday use of our bodies and come to assume a habitus that expresses our tastes or preferences for various goods, including symbolic goods. In the process of this embodiment, we also develop a capacity for self-reflection that is always expressed through embodiment. Our selfhood is reflected in the peculiarities of our own embodiment; our eccentricity is articulated through these bodily practices and our habitus. Two processes – embodiment and what I call enselfment – express the idea that mind and body are never separated. Who we are is a social process that is always constructed in terms of a particular experience of embodiment. Suffering (the loss of dignity) and pain (a loss of comfort) are always intertwined, and so vulnerability is both a physical and spiritual condition. Finally, our experience of the everyday world involves a particular place – a location within which experiences of the body and our dependency on other humans unfold. The notion of emplacement is taken from Heidegger's (1962) account of *Being and Time* in which the concept *Dasein*, or literally 'there-being', specifies the temporality of being. Heidegger's philosophy of being-in-time conceptualized the inevitable contingency of human existence. Given the ineluctable contingency of the everyday world, 'emplacement' is crucial for our sense of identity, security and continuity. Human beings need comfort in order to experience security, certainty and confidence. As a result, human-rights violations typically involve some attack on the body through torture and deprivation, an assault on the dignity of the self through psychological damage, and some disruption to place through exclusion and displacement (imprisonment, deportation, seizure of land and exile). Human rights abuses disrupt, disconnect and destroy the very conditions that make embodiment, enselfment and emplacement possible. Given this intimate connection between self, body and habitus, it is difficult to see how immortality could be achieved, for example, through cryonics without losing our identity. To preserve my identity, I not only need my memory to be intact, but I need to be able to recreate my habitus, my social network and my unique form of embodiment.

The vulnerability of our everyday world is connected to a sociological understanding of the precarious nature of institutions. We need to understand the social world in terms of the relationship between these two processes: embodiment and institutionalization. In sociological theory, 'institutions' replace 'instincts', because human beings do not have many ready-made instinctual responses to their environment. Human instincts are malleable, minimal and non-specific. Hence, human society involves the building of an infinite number of institutions – courtship, the family, religion, rituals, eating patterns, sleeping arrangements and political ceremonials. 'Institutions' are patterns of social interaction that are sustained by customs and sanctions. Learning to live in society means learning how these institutions work – or do not work. We create institutions in order to have security, thereby reducing our vulnerability, but these institutional patterns are always imperfect, inadequate and precarious. The point is to develop a general sociology of everyday life based on the concepts of embodiment, institutions and social connectedness that in turn lay the foundation for the study of human rights that are institutional manifestations of our social dependency. This discussion of vulnerability and rights has to be located within a global context, where the hybridity and fragmentation of culture brings into question our capacity to sustain solidarity in the everyday world.

The idea of vulnerable humanity recognizes the obviously corporeal dimension of existence; it describes the condition of sentient, embodied creatures, who are exposed to the dangers of their environment, and who are conscious of their precarious circumstances. This theme of human vulnerability clearly has strong religious connotations. In mediaeval religious practice and belief, veneration of the Passion was associated with meditation on the Seven Wounds of Christ. Our vulnerability is a wounding that is traumatic; it signifies the capacity to be open to wounding, and to be open to the world. In modern usage, the notion of vulnerability has become, in one sense, more abstract; it refers to human openness to psychological harm or moral damage or spiritual threat. It refers increasingly to our ability to suffer psychologically, morally and spiritually rather than simply to a physical capacity for pain from our exposure to the world.

As an aspect of human frailty, our vulnerability includes the idea that human beings of necessity have an organic propensity to disease and sickness, that death and dying are inescapable, and that our ageing bodies are subject to impairment and disability. The traditional human life cycle was characterized by its finite possibilities, and hence it was seen to be inescapably tragic. As a result of these traditional conditions, human beings have been, through their life cycle, involved in various relationships of dependency. Arnold Gehlen (1988) employed Nietzsche's aphorism that we are 'unfinished animals' to develop an anthropological view of the frailty of human beings. Given this incompleteness, human beings need to build institutions to compensate, as it were, for their biological lack of instincts. Human beings are characterized by their 'instinctual deprivation' and as a result they do not have a stable structure within which to operate. Humans are also defined by their 'world openness', because they are not equipped instinctively for a specific environment, and as a result they have to build or construct their own social environment, a construction that requires the building of institutions. Social institutions are the bridges between humans and their physical environment, and it is through these institutions that human life becomes coherent, meaningful and continuous (Berger and Kellner 1965). In filling the gap created by instinctual deprivation, institutions provide humans with psychological relief from the tensions generated by undirected instinctual drives.

The normative order (*nomos*) that human societies construct in response to the absence of specific functional instincts constitutes a social shelter or 'sacred canopy' (Berger 1967). We can elaborate Berger's sociology of religion to develop the idea that, as part of the protective environment of world-open human beings, legal institutions are fundamental in providing some degree of security in this precarious environment. It is possible to derive the basic forms of a juridical canopy, in terms of the rule of law – habeas corpus, civil liberties and rights – from this account of the ontological incompleteness of humans. From this basic philosophical account, human rights can be seen as a component of this protective juridical shield, in which the social canopy is constructed of both rites (sacred institutions) and rights (legal devices of security).

## Institution Building

This construction of institutions is not necessarily a self-conscious or reflective activity, and indeed these social arrangements have to have a certain taken-for-granted character. Where such institutions become traditional, they are part of the taken-for-granted back-cloth of social relations that makes everyday social action possible. These traditional, background assumptions give social life a certain degree of social stability and psychological security. Where the background is traditional, the foreground is by contrast occupied by more reflexive, practical and conscious activities. With modernization, there is a process of deinstitutionalization with the result that the background assumptions of social action become, in subjective terms, less reliable and tangible, more open to negotiation and increasingly, objects of critical and rational reflection. Accordingly, the unstable foreground expands, and life becomes more risky and precarious. The objective and sacred institutions of tradition recede, and modern life becomes risky, unstable and uncertain. Modernization involves a reflective increase in the flexibility of norms and institutions that change constantly in response to the pace of social change. In fact, we live in a world of what Gehlen called secondary or quasi-institutions.

There are profound psychological consequences associated with these changes. Human beings in archaic societies had 'character', i.e., a firm and definite psychological structure that corresponded to reliable background institutions. In modern societies, the individual has become a 'personality', living in a 'lonely crowd' (Riesman 1950) and thus, people come to have personalities that are fluid and flexible, like the uncertain and fluid institutions in which they live. We can argue in these terms that the modernization of societies involves a 'foregrounding' of cultural practices and institutions that can no longer be taken for granted. With the modern medical science revolution, the ageing cycle can no longer be taken for granted and age and death are both redefined. The expansion of life expectancy has transformed death, and patients can be sustained by medical technology for an indefinite period. These developments constitute a radical assault on conventional religious notions about desire, worldliness and heaven. St Augustine sharply distinguished two powerful human desires: *cupiditas* (or the desire for worldly goods) and *caritas* (or the love of God that is manifest in the virtue of charity). Human life is a constant, and largely unsuccessful, struggle to overcome the sins of the flesh as manifest most powerfully in greed (Kent 2001). The unity of virtue in charity is the condition, not the object, of goodness. This Christian notion of virtue, which Augustine developed from traditional Greek philosophy, has a very uncertain location in a world where life might, in principle, continue indefinitely.

Contemporary theories of social risk suggest that modern social systems cannot effectively resolve the complexities and contingencies of social change, cultural diversity, environmental pollution and urban decay and hence, institutional precariousness is a function of modernization, i.e., a function of the globalization of risk (Beck 2000). In turn, human vulnerability is also increased, despite the important historical success of public-health movements, improvements in healthcare, and various spectacular breakthroughs in medical science, such as vaccination. This dynamic relationship between institutional precariousness and human vulnerability is the driver of the evolution of human rights legislation and culture. Institutions need to be continuously repaired and redesigned, and human rights need to be constantly reviewed in the light of their misapplication, misappropriation and failures. In short, the aim of this theory is to give a dynamic account of the relationship between the human condition and institution building.

Both of these arguments (vulnerability and precariousness) are an attempt to develop a contemporary version of Hobbes's theory of the state without the limitations of a utilitarian and rational theory of social contract based on self-interest. Hobbes (2003) argued in *Leviathan* that rational human beings with conflicting interests in a state of nature would be in a condition of perpetual war. In order to protect themselves from mutual, endless slaughter, they create a state in the basis of a social contract, which organizes society in the collective interest of rational but antagonistic and competitive human beings. Furthermore, the institutions, which humans create as protective or defensive mechanisms, have to be sufficiently powerful to regulate an individualistic market society, and as a consequence the state can develop as a political agency that is necessarily a threat to human beings. For example, the state, which holds a monopoly over legalized violence, is both a guarantor of social security and an instrument, necessarily, of violence. The internationalization of human rights is intended to act as a check on state power and to guarantee that states respect the rights of their citizens. The problem is to create international agencies that can (morally and legally) coerce states.

## Some Objections to the Vulnerability Argument

The argument that embodiment is a fruitful basis for the defence the universalism of human rights is based on the notion of the ubiquity of human suffering. In 1850 Arthur Schopenhauer (2004) opened his essay 'On the Suffering of the World' with the observation that every 'individual misfortune, to be sure, seems an exceptional occurrence; but misfortune in general is the rule.' While the study of misery and misfortune has been the stuff of philosophy and theology, there is little systematic study of these phenomena by sociologists. One exception is Barrington Moore (1970, 11) who argues in *Reflections on the Causes of Human Misery* that 'suffering is not a value in its own right. In this sense any form of suffering becomes a cost, and unnecessary suffering an odious cost. Similarly, general opposition to human suffering constitutes a standpoint that both transcends and unites different cultures and historical epochs.' A critic might object that suffering is too variable in its cultural manifestations and too vague in its meanings to provide the moral basis for such a common standpoint. What actually constitutes human suffering might well turn out to be, in cultural terms, highly specific. Those who take note of the cultural variability of suffering have, for example, made similar arguments against a common standard of disability. Although one could well accept this anthropological argument on the grounds that suffering involves essentially the devaluation of a person as a consequence of accident, affliction or torture, pain is less historically and socially variable. Whereas bankruptcy, for instance, would involve some degree of variable psychological suffering, a toothache is a toothache. If we claim that disability is a social condition (the loss of social rights) and thus relative, we might reasonably argue that impairment is the underlying condition about which there is less political dispute. In short, some conditions or states of affairs are less socially constructed than others are. Pain is less variable than suffering, if we regard the latter as a form of indignity. In most human societies, suffering is closely associated with ageing, since it is in the ageing process that we most profoundly experience the inconvenience of physical immobility, an erosion of our dignity and the decline of our social status. Ageing in this regard most clearly illustrates our vulnerability, partly because it ultimately robs us of our autonomy and exposes us to conditions over which we no longer have control. Before the modern revolution in medical sciences, the experience of ageing and its associated disability was the common experience of humanity. The life extension project brings these assumptions into question and, if successful, promises to undermine those common experiences of decline.

There is a strong argument, then, in support of the existence of a community of sentiment determined by the negative consequences of pain and suffering, which are clearly leading indicators of human vulnerability. This notion that there can be a cross-cultural understanding of the bond of suffering was perfectly expressed in Shakespeare's *The Merchant of Venice* where Shylock in Act III scene 1 offers a challenge to the standard forms of Elizabethan anti-Semitism: 'If you prick us do we not bleed?' The experience of vulnerability provides a norm for the assertion of a human bond across generations and cultures, and this cross-cultural characteristic of vulnerability presupposes the embodiment of the human agent. A moral and political philosophy that is closely connected with the notions of embodiment, suffering and justice, was powerfully developed in Mahatma Gandhi's struggle to control rising ethnic and religious conflict between Muslims and Hindus in the context of Indian postcolonialism. Gandhi's commitment to simplicity and nonviolence was deeply rooted in Hindu culture, but it also drew inspiration from western, specifically German, naturopathy, which in turn entailed a critique of the rationalist and mechanistic assumptions of allopathic, Western and colonial medicine. Gandhi's development of a government of the body or control of the senses (*brahmacharya*) was intended to give individuals and social movements the power to resist colonial occupation and to transcend physical pollution and political corruption. Gandhi's philosophical defence of peaceful struggle provides further ammunition for the notion that vulnerability is the underlying foundation of respect for others, and his openness to heterogeneous philosophical sources indicates that, with globalization, assumptions about local, autonomous cultures are questionable. We need, therefore, to understand this vulnerability against a background of global risks that in turn draw attention to the precarious nature of human institutions.

Perhaps the major criticism of this vulnerability argument is the medical technology paradox. The more medical science improves our health condition, the less vulnerable we are. Therefore, technological progress could make this vulnerability thesis historically specific. In principle, if we live longer because we have become less vulnerable with technological advances, then the relevance of human rights might diminish. This paradox helps me to sharpen my argument, which is that we are human because we are vulnerable. We could only finally escape our vulnerability by ultimately escaping from our own humanity. Technological progress promises to create a posthuman world in which, with medical progress, we could, in principle, live forever. This criticism is a very interesting argument, but there are two potentially important counterarguments. The first is that if we could increase our life expectancy, then we would live longer, but with higher rates of morbidity and disability. The quantity of life might increase in years, but there would be a corresponding decline in its quality. A posthuman world is a medical utopia that has all the negative features of a Brave New World. Whether modern science can ultimately solve the Tithonus Fallacy by giving us both longevity and rejuvenation remains to be seen. It is unlikely that the medical interventions necessary to keep us young can be available to everyone. Secondly, medical improvements in the advanced societies are likely to increase the inequality between societies, creating a more unequal and insecure international order. In such a risk society, where human precariousness increased and human vulnerability decreased, the need for human rights protection would continue. The prospect of living forever might require us to inhabit, in Max Weber's pessimistic metaphor, a biological 'iron cage' in which our existence was by courtesy of life-support machines. But can this Brave New World overcome what I will refer to as 'natural scarcity' and hence replace the need for rationing such scarce resources?

## Ageing, Healthcare and Longevity

Perhaps the acid test of arguments about longevity, vulnerability and justice is whether we can justify the allocation of scarce health resources in support of the elderly. I have already raised the issue of intergenerational justice in Chapter Four, and in the following chapter on social rights I will consider Aubrey de Grey's argument that we have a right to life. But are these rights to be shared equally by different age groups in a context of rising health costs? Where there is scarcity, there is normally some principle of queuing in which goods and services are allocated. Given the fact that the demand on health services is heavily skewed towards those over 75 years of age, what principles of justice might apply if we are to care for the elderly? There are two issues here. As a matter of fact people are living longer and hence there is an immediate and vexed policy issue about the allocation of health resources that might be consistent with an ethic of care towards the elderly. There is the additional issue relating to Immortalism. If de Grey's vision of rejuvenated longevity were to become a reality, what are the economic and moral implications for healthcare? Furthermore, could we justify the investment in geriatric research that will be necessary to bring this geriatric utopia into existence?

Many of the policy and philosophical issues of the economics of rationing on the basis of age have been extensively discussed by Ian Dey and Neil Fraser (2000) in their valuable article on 'Age-Based Rationing in the Allocation of Health Care'. I shall outline their argument and the attempt to examine the extra complications that are presented by the hypothetical utopia of a society of immortals. The point of this exercise is that it exposes very clearly that the Immortalists have not seriously considered the economics of prolongevity, but more importantly, the issue of justice in healthcare brings out the deeply individualistic nature of their thought. Dey and Fraser's general conclusion is that age does not provide a useful or just criterion for resource allocation, but they recognize that some form of age-related allocation is likely to remain a feature of healthcare systems. If age does function in decisions about resource allocation, it should be overt and transparent rather than covert and obscure.

The traditional welfare state has been heavily criticized from the perspective of neoliberal economics. The arguments in favour of individual responsibility and privatization have been reinforced by arguments pointing out that the ageing of populations will put an intolerable burden on universalistic welfare because of an adverse dependency ratio and because of an erosion of the tax basis of society. This analysis is often coupled with the view that expenditure on the health needs of the elderly reduces the resources available for younger age groups. For example Callahan (1987) called for a shift in the allocation of resources away from the elderly in favour of younger generations. Dey and Fraser explore the principles that might be and in many cases are already involved in making practical, transparent and justifiable decisions about health resource allocation on the basis of age. They start their examination by suggesting that there are four levels at which rationing decisions might be undertaken. The first is the societal level where governments might attempt to develop policy statements about age-related entitlement. Secondly, there is a strategic level in which health authorities may be given responsibility to decide on resource allocation. Thirdly, there may be a pragmatic level in which screening programmes are judged at an institutional level in terms of their effectiveness. Finally, there is a clinical level in which doctors or nurses make decisions based on covert values and assumptions about which patients might get what type of treatment. They argue, reasonably, that such clinical decisions are likely to be covert and in many cases arbitrary and prejudicial.

In the next stage of their argument, they suggest that decisions about resource allocation might be made according to three criteria: effectiveness, efficiency and fairness. In general they argue that many of the measures of effectiveness and efficiency are unreliable and often biased against the elderly. For example, QALYs (Quality-Adjusted Life-Years) are often used to measure effectiveness. One major issue with modern medicine is that doctors are often more concerned to experiment with new methods that may be costly, involving intrusive technological interventions, but offer patients relatively little experience of enhanced quality of life. QALYs may discriminate against a patient who is, for example, 75 years of age where a medical intervention is assessed on the health benefits over a period of five or ten years. The use of QALYs reflects a utilitarian philosophy of achieving the greatest benefit for the greatest number, but they cannot tell us whose health condition should be maximized. Is it better to save six QALYs for one person or five

QALYs for five people? This issue in fact raises a more profound problem, which is that expenditure on people who are profoundly disabled would not be supported by the use of QALYs as a criterion, since their prospects of improvement are low by comparison with somebody whose condition can be cured. Furthermore, if the elderly are seen to be a burden on healthcare systems, perhaps we should allocate resources by taking gender into account. Because women have a longer life expectancy, critics would have to recommend discriminating against women.

One argument that has gained support is the notion, based upon a cricketing metaphor, that the elderly have already enjoyed a 'fair innings' and therefore it is only reasonable to favour younger age groups in any situation of scarcity. This notion has become central to most debates about equity. Given the constraints on modern healthcare systems, it is argued that since the elderly have already enjoyed the allocation of resources in their lifetime, benefits should go to the young to secure a lifetime experience of health. The fair innings argument is supported by the notion that life has a natural course with a definite ending and that everybody shares, more or less, in this ageing process. It would be unreasonable to allocate resources to the elderly in a context where their natural life cannot be extended indefinitely. It is this assumption of a natural life course that the life extension programme wants to challenge. We might note, therefore, that the fair innings argument might not apply where life was being extended indefinitely.

Regardless of these philosophical arguments, we know as a matter of fact that at the clinical level nurses and doctors discriminate on the basis of age. In many areas of medicine – renal failure, coronary attacks, hypertension and certain cancers – decisions based on age are routine, albeit covert (Kapp 1998). Social factors persistently influence medical decision-making. In both private and public health services, 'the sophisticated, the wealthy, and the powerful almost always find their way to the head of the rationing line' (Goodman and Musgrave 1992, xx). One limitation with much of this discussion in medical ethics is that it appears to ignore social class differences between patients, and also differences between healthcare systems that have been largely privatized. If the wealthy elderly can pay for their privileged position at the head of the queue, who are we to say they should not be there? One argument would be that because the distribution of wealth in society is not strictly related to merit (intelligence or hard work), but more related to the arbitrary outcome of inheritance, the wealthy do not deserve to be at the head of the queue. However, the problem with the free market and the contemporary emphasis on deregulation and market-driven criteria is that markets and virtues have become separated. But can a civilized society be based on these market values without falling into a Darwinian survival of the fittest? Blatant inequalities in healthcare, for example, depending on one's postal address in the United Kingdom are regarded as offensive in a democracy where there are social rights to equality in healthcare.

As a set of principles, discrimination and rationing by age are not promising foundations for healthcare. Most of the cost of caring for the elderly comes at the very end of life. As compulsory retirement disappears, the elderly may continue with gainful employment well into old age, making a valuable contribution to society. Furthermore, scarcity is not a neutral category, since much of the scarcity in public provision is a consequence of government decisions about national priorities. Nevertheless, age is a basis for what I have called 'moral queuing', i.e., a queue based upon a moral judgement as opposed to the idea of first come, first served. Dey and Fraser (2000, 534) conclude that, at the clinical level, 'the covert use of age in limiting treatment is routinely justified in terms of (clinical) assessment of needs, even though the evidence strongly suggests that practitioners often discriminate by age independently of individual functioning or capacity to benefit.' In terms of the cricketing metaphor, who is to say that a fair innings comes to an end when you have your half-century or your century? At what point does the capacity of an individual to contribute to society appear to have been eclipsed? This issue raises a related question, which is whether there should be a right to die for people who are suffering from painful, humiliating and ultimately terminable illness. Indeed, is there a duty to die? (Battin, 1987).

## Conclusion: Vulnerability and Virtue

In contemporary social theory, Paul Rabinow (1996) and Nikolas Rose (2001) have argued that we are currently witnessing a radical and total transformation in the organization of embodied life.

Against the idea that life is fixed, Rabinow and Rose draw upon contemporary biomedicine to argue that life is malleable and can be assembled out of a variety of biomolecular components. Modern politics is about 'life itself' and the new medical technologies open up new opportunities for increasing the productivity and efficiency of life. These arguments are persuasive, but for the time being and for the great majority of human beings, the experiences of life and death are relatively unchanged. The majority of human beings, for the foreseeable future, will experience the diseases of old age in our final years. From the perspective of phenomenology, the experience of death in a modern hospital is not wholly unlike the experience of death of our grandparents. What has changed radically is the understanding of old age and death, and this new understanding has significant implications for longevity. In terms of modern biomedicine, as we saw in chapter one, Thomas Kirkwood's definition of ageing as the failure to sustain adequate investments in cellular repair provides a critical way of thinking about ageing in terms of the balance between the organism's maintenance and germinal continuity. Life becomes a trade-off around the investments required by reproduction and the continuity of germinal trays. We can refine my notion of vulnerability as the mortality and finitude of somatic lines in contrast to the immortality of the germinal lines. The great evolutionary biologists of ageing on whom the modern science of microbiology rests – Weismann, Hayflick and Kirkwood – recognized that there is another set of investments that are important, namely, the social investments in sustaining and protecting an elderly population. Therefore, our vulnerability is a function of two forms of investment – in repairing damaged cells and in sustaining social institutions. We are biologically vulnerable as a result of damage to cells and socially vulnerable as a result of damage to institutions.

*Vulnerability and Human Rights* (Turner 2006a) developed the idea that our humanity rests on our vulnerability, i.e., our capacity to be wounded. Because humans are vulnerable, they need an array of social rights to give them some basic security just to exist. These institutions we build are however themselves precarious and hence our security will always involve an ongoing contingent struggle to provide some safety net of rights and laws.

By entering the debate on human rights via the idea of human vulnerability, I considered both physical and mental vulnerability.

In modern advanced societies it may be that we have partly solved the issue of physical vulnerability – rising life expectancy is demonstrable proof of this success – but we are a long way from solving mental vulnerability, as measured by mental illness, drug dependency, unhappiness and a sense of meaninglessness that are so characteristic of modern society. Much of the literature suggests that in a consumer society there is a negative correlation between personal happiness and rising per capita incomes. More significantly, I think there is a spiritual vacuum in modern societies that no medical advance can satisfy.

Precisely because man's life is nasty, brutish and short, we need strong institutions to secure even a minimal level of civilized life, and we find that these arrangements are constantly breaking down. Human beings have responded to this problem by developing institutions and technology to cope with our natural precariousness. I want to argue that in order for human beings to cope with vulnerability they are obviously from childhood dependent on adults for what sociologists call 'socialization', i.e., to become adults and citizens they need long periods of training and education simply to function effectively in society. But this idea of 'socialization' does not adequately capture the notion that to be human at all, people need to enjoy and to enjoy successfully a life-long experience of being nurtured. This is the conventional argument against socialization – it does not refer only to childhood, but to the life process.

From feminist theory, we are familiar with the idea that care and nurturing are critical prerequisites of the development of mature personalities and that without this ongoing care we cannot really be equipped to become ethical creatures. Without a sense of being nurtured, and hence, being wanted by another human being, I cannot become an adult capable of respecting other human beings. To be nurtured provides me with the capacities that I need in order to nurture somebody else. In short I have, as a defenceless child, a right to be nurtured or cared for and hence, I have a duty to respect other people and to care for them.

We normally express these issues in terms of intergenerational justice when we come to express how I have a responsibility to pass on to the next generation the resources and advantages that I have received in the process of growing up. But these rights and duties should not be expressed in terms of filial piety – these are duties I have towards fellow human beings. The point of this argument is that I cannot nurture unless I have been nurtured, and I cannot be ethically responsible unless I am in some sort of caring relationship.

This idea of nurturing strikes me as a useful way of extending the original idea of vulnerability as a method of avoiding cultural relativism and as a way of providing the basis for claims regarding social rights. Thus the *Oxford English Dictionary* draws our attention to the common roots of the verbs to nurse, to nurture and to nourish. Feeding the body as the right to nourishment might also imply, therefore, not only the right to be nurtured and nourished in order to become fully human as an ethical agent, but also the duties we all carry as a result of previous nourishment, however inadequate and limited.

This approach raises all sorts of problems about gender, care and responsibility, especially responsibility to children, and the differentiation of male and female roles. For example, this argument about nourishment obviously raises issues about the place of family life, motherhood and fatherhood in human societies and about the rights of reproduction. Article 16 of the United Nations Universal Declaration of Human Rights says that men and women of full age 'have the right to marry and to found a family'.

This may provide a useful point at which to try to answer the question: What might a sociology of human rights look like? Most of the answers so far are implicitly that sociology, in taking a critical view of individualism as a modern ideology, concerns itself with the origin, nature and defence of the social rights that are only partially embedded in existing human rights declarations and thinking. What I am suggesting here is that by looking at reproduction, sociology might draw attention to the ethic of care – nurturing, nourishing and nursing – that is so central to the production of fully rounded human beings as agents capable also of caring, and hence, of exercising responsibility, and to all of those institutions that relate to caring such as motherhood, nursing, families, schools and other communal arrangements.

One solution to this issue could be drawn from the theory of human capacities in the work of Amartya Sen and Martha Nussbaum, and especially in Nussbaum's recent work on *Frontiers of Justice* (Nussbaum 2006). The capabilities model puts human development (including care and nourishment) at the centre of any discussion of human rights and justice, but it also recognizes that the satisfaction of human needs (nourishment and shelter) cannot be achieved outside a process of democratization. This conclusion goes back to Sen's economic arguments that, for example, no democracy has experienced a famine – i.e., famine is a function of inadequate resource management and massive inequality in the distribution of resources. Therefore, we cannot artificially separate arguments that defend individual rights from arguments that defend social rights.

Our vulnerability in old age is not simply physical; it is exacerbated by the loss of friends and hence, the loss of care and personal nourishment. The loneliness of the elderly is a basic cause of depression and poor health. Elderly old men in inner cities areas are especially vulnerable in this respect (Klinenberg 2002). However, caring or nourishing cannot be entirely one-way. To nourish is also to be nourished. Unfortunately, there is no simple cure for the unhappiness that the elderly experience in their isolation. The happiness tablets that Immortalists promise us may be simply a repeat of the history of the failure of Prozac.

Why is it that it takes one a lifetime to recognize and to realize these simple truths? One answer is that before we enter into the slow march towards old age, we live through a period of our lives that is characterized by what I will call the arrogance of invincibility in which ageing and death can make no appearance. Youth has the illusion of invincibility.

# Chapter Seven

## Towards a New Paradigm of Ageing

### Introduction: The Rights Discourse

I started this book with the debate between optimists such as Paine, Godwin and Condorcet and pessimists such as Malthus and Ricardo over the prospects for happiness and a full life, especially as it had been envisaged by Paine (1995) in his *Rights of Man*. While prolongevity obviously raises factual problems about the feasibility of life extension such as freezing whole bodies, it very definitely raises ethical and philosophical problems about how life extension might be justified. In this book I am claiming that there are two important frameworks for its justification. One is an aesthetic justification, which I am deriving from Nietzsche, that by making our lives into a work of art we might justify long life both to ourselves and to others. The alternative is justification in terms of rights (either human rights or the social rights of citizenship). In this rights framework, the right to long life might be developed as fundamentally an extension of a right to life as such or a right to health. Let us turn again to the question of rights.

Egalitarian concepts of social justice and human rights have been used in diverse ways in the life extension project debate. Researchers who are sympathetic to the project have both drawn upon and rejected the egalitarian approach in their argumentation. Generally speaking, they highlight the untenable position of delaying scientific progress while governments and international agencies attempt to resolve existing problems of global social inequality (Post 2004). Hence, these scientific benefits are perceived to outweigh the various social challenges that are brought about by rejuvenation research (Stock and Callahan 2004). In contrast, by supporting the rejuvenation sciences, posthumanist thinking has drawn on egalitarianism to protect the social rights of older adults through interventions in the ageing process. The main thrust of this perspective is to reduce negative ageism, providing equal opportunities for older adults to achieve optimal longevity (by delaying or preventing death). The following quotation clearly illustrates a radical form of anti-ageism:

> ...the popular view that saving lives of children in Africa (for example) is more important than curing aging constitutes discrimination in favor of those whose remaining lives will be very short unless we help them but fairly short even if we do, and against those who will probably live a few decades anyway but could live many centuries if we act now [...] Thus, to prioritize expenditure on treating diseases of old age... and to deprioritize expenditure on curing aging constitutes discrimination against those just young enough to benefit from a cure for aging if we threw more resources now at developing it.
>
> (de Grey 2004c, 166)

The pursuit of scientific progress and the perception of injustice towards the right of the elderly to sufficient biomedical expenditure in rejuvenation sciences require a response. There may be a right to adequate healthcare for the elderly, but it is clearly too simplistic to accept the full autonomy of biogerontologists who want to increase longevity without considering its negative consequences (Hayflick 2000). Indeed, rejuvenation research will affect politics through the prolongation of life and a series of demographic and social changes will eventually occur as a consequence (Fukuyama 2002). These consequences will be the result primarily of the uneven and unequal global distribution of economic and social resources.

In traditional societies, the relationship between resources, especially the food supply, and life expectancy was, more or less, regulated by a Malthusian logic. Although demographic history has not fully supported this Malthusian pessimism, it is self-evident that powerful groups would benefit more than others from the life extension technology. If we assume that, while medical sciences could reduce mortality, they would, at least in the short term, increase morbidity as chronic illness and geriatric diseases increased. Life extension would mean, in practice, living longer in discomfort, i.e., in a morbid condition. There would therefore have to be increasing investment in resources to solve physiological (chronic illnesses) and psychological problems (depression, ennui and despair). De Grey's argument is that rejuvenation can solve these problems by managing morbidity more effectively, but this rejuvenation project remains a long-term objective.

The UN Universal Declaration of Human Rights has much to say, as one might imagine, about life. For example, Article 3 proclaims that 'Everyone has the right to life, liberty and security of person', and other articles refer to the right to freedom from torture. Article 16 includes 'the right to marry and to found a family' and Article 25 talks about 'the right to a standard of living adequate for health and well-being . . .' There are many conceptual problems with this list of rights in the Declaration. In the literature there is much confusion about the rights of humans as humans and the rights of citizens as members of a polity; sometimes this distinction is conceptualized as the difference between the individual rights of people as human beings and the social rights of members of a collectivity. Whereas we might say that all human beings have a right to life regardless of their social membership, Article 22 refers more specifically to the entitlements of citizens when it proclaims that 'Everyone, as a member of a society, has the right to social security . . .' Does this imply a right to live forever?

## Justification of Longevity by a Rights Discourse

In an interview with de Grey, Sherwin Nuland, in the *Technological Review* of February 2005, challenged de Grey to provide justification for his longevity programme. In the course of presenting his question, Nuland provided a list of the implications of the SENS programme that are worth listing here. The issues include: the huge investment of scientific research funding; the transformation of human culture from a limited lifespan to an indefinite one; the fact that every human being could, in principle, be the same physiological age following mass rejuvenation programmes; and the effect on family relations. De Grey's answer was that people have a human right to live as long as they can; as an extension of the idea of a duty of care, people have a right to expect to be treated as they would treat themselves; and finally, scientists have a duty to develop these therapies as quickly as possible to give future generations this choice. These rights claims are derived, in his view, from the basic religious and moral standpoint that the right to life is the most important right of all.

Before we can tackle these issues directly, we need to draw attention again to a problem that, in my view, is generic to de Grey's argument. If we make a distinction between what we might call 'mere existence' and 'life', then it makes little sense to ask whether we have a right to existence (either prolonged or otherwise). As a member of the human species, it makes little sense for me to ask: Do I have a right to exist? My existence, like the existence of other creatures, is simply a fact of history. I simply am. As a creature, rights and duties do not, as such, impinge on my mere existence. Whereas mere existence is the fact of being alive, life is the full panoply of my culture, language, social relations, consciousness, memory and human dignity. It does make sense, therefore, to ask whether I have a right to life and secondly, whether I have a right to extend it without limit. I shall argue further that this right to life only becomes intelligible if one can outline what the duties relating to prolongevity might be. Legal scholars often argue that there has to be 'correlativity' between rights and duties. If I have a right to free speech, it implies duties to protect that right to a voice, to defend the integrity of journalism and to defend a democratic civil sphere in which there is a free flow of communication. The relationship between rights and duties is never exact, but we might argue that a strong notion of right carries with it a definite conception of duty. The immediate task is therefore to outline a political framework in which one could justify life extension by reference to a cluster of duties. A right to life implies a duty to future generations to secure for them, as far as possible, the same opportunities and conditions that my generation has enjoyed during its lifespan. One can immediately see the problem of intergenerational justice in the Immortalist framework. If, after the discovery of the full range of rejuvenative medicine, my generation does not pass away, then it is difficult to see how this exchange of resources could take place.

One immediate objection, therefore, to de Grey is the following: Throughout the twentieth century there has been a great inflation of human rights claims, some of which are not feasible and many are fanciful. There is a general tendency towards rights inflation taking place with no correlative development of the idea of a duty. It is relatively easy to claim a right, but we need more solid grounds to justify such claims. Prolongevity at the very least implies a decline of resources, if one accepts the standard economic arguments about scarcity.

Where did this right to life come from? The Universal Declaration of Human Rights was written in 1948 in the aftermath of the Second World War when its primary concern was to counteract the consequences of the devastation that had been wrought on civilian populations. Since the victims of modern warfare were primarily civilians and not combatants, human rights established new principles to cope with the victims of technological mass warfare. Neither the possibility nor the desirability that medical science could significantly prolong life was on the agenda of politicians and lawmakers in the late 1940s. However, coming towards the end of a long consumer boom in the late twentieth and early twenty-first centuries, the issue of whether there might be a right to prolong life indefinitely is now on the horizon of various think tanks, scientific institutions and utopian social movements. The question of a right to indefinitely prolonged life needs attention philosophically, legally and sociologically. Whether life can be significantly prolonged is still contentious, but the ageing of the world's population does, as a matter of fact, as we have noted in previous chapters, raise important questions about the equal distribution of natural resources. This demographic transition brings into focus the particular issue of the rights of children that are part of intergenerational justice, but it is difficult to conceptualize living forever within the conventional paradigm of human rights.

The Declaration does not obviously or explicitly say that we have a right to live forever or merely for as long as possible. But in declaring that we have rights to 'health and well-being', it could be reasonably interpreted as implying at least that the aspiration to live long, healthy and satisfactory lives is a rational and justifiable aspiration. Is there a right to health or only a right to healthcare? Living forever implies adequate healthcare and resources to fund the range of medical interventions that are contained with the rejuvenation dreams of de Grey, Dexler, Kurzweil and others. I want to argue that a right to healthcare can only make sense in the context of a nation state that undertakes to provide its citizens with care. The notion of a right to healthcare in the universalistic framework of human rights does not look meaningful, let alone feasible, since it is not clear who will offer these health services globally. The UN has neither the capacity nor the mandate. Human rights and other international agencies tend to offer healthcare in response to an emergency such as a tsunami, but providing healthcare over the long term to the elderly, for example, is typically undertaken within the framework of a national welfare state or at least a welfare system that plugs the gaps created by declining family structures or inadequate private provision. It is difficult to suggest that we possess, by virtue of being human beings, a right to long life on the basis of a comprehensive healthcare system. When human rights were framed within the Declaration, the implicit assumption was probably that good health was a contingent outcome of genetics, education and good fortune. Good health is not something for which one can legislate. Health appears to be more the consequence of accident rather than design. In addition to the genetic legacy we inherit from our parents, our health, in modern Britain for example, depends on a range of contingent factors: our social class and income level, the quality of healthcare in the region in which we live and the doctor–patient ratio, our gender, our educational attainment and many local circumstances (water quality, housing stock and environmental hazard from power stations). Health depends significantly on lifestyle (our diet) and on sheer natural good fortune (our height, for example) (Turner 2004). In fact, health is, in practice, defined not in a positive fashion, but in residual terms as the absence of sickness and disease. While we might have an abstract right to healthcare, whether that right can be institutionalized depends on a range of contingent conditions. The complexity of the causes of good health reaffirms the criticism that prolongevity will only be, and can only be, available to an affluent and powerful elite. It may be that we do not have a right to healthcare, but, more realistically, an expectation that the inequalities that are associated with sickness and disease would be minimized by public-health measures and social investment.

There is, furthermore, as I have indicated, a fundamental problem about the validity of the discourse of rights and duties itself. In response to the American and French Revolutions that inaugurated the modern language of universal rights, many British politicians and philosophers declared these rights to be nonsensical. Edmund Burke claimed that the actual rights of an Englishman (as a member of a state) were more concrete and effective than the abstract, fanciful 'rights of Man'. In his *Anarchical Fallacies*, Jeremy Bentham declared that the idea of 'natural and imprescriptible rights' was 'nonsense on stilts' (Waldron 1987). The point of the ideological battle between Paine and Lafayette on the one hand, and Burke and Bentham on the other, was that human rights could only be implemented by sovereign (nation) states and therefore 'the rights of Man' would be in reality dependent upon 'the rights of the citizen'. For many modern commentators, this situation has not changed. Only sovereign states can protect the human rights of individuals (Birmingham 2006).

We need to clarify whether a right to life can be housed within a human rights discourse or whether it pertains more significantly to the social rights of citizens living within a political community or state. The problem of individual rights – or *my* right to life extension – is related to individualism, namely, whether the rational desire to extend my life is compatible with the needs of the community, i.e., with collective rights. If one accepts the assumption of classical political economy (such as Malthus) that human beings cannot escape scarcity, then any (indefinite) extension of life will have serious consequences for collective resources and especially for how those resources are distributed over time. Does a significant extension of my life reduce the resources available to the social group, thereby constraining the rights of others to enjoy a modicum of healthcare?

Modern citizenship has historically been constructed around a set of contributory rights and duties that are related to work, public service (for example, military or jury service) and parenthood or family formation. It defines membership of a society through the entitlements that are associated with service, and is perhaps most clearly evident in a national system of taxation or in conscription into the army (Turner 1993). This model of citizenship as contributory social rights has been closely associated with the legacy of the English sociologist Thomas H. Marshall (1893–1982). Marshallian citizenship has been subject to considerable criticism over the last two decades and the social model of citizenship has been expanded and deepened by approaches that emphasize the flexibility of social membership, the limitations of citizenship merely as contributory rights and by perspectives that emphasise identity and difference. This early model of citizenship has been considerably extended to include many new forms of social rights such as sexual, green and environmental citizenship. The latter might, for example, include the right of citizens to have clean air. Environmental citizenship may well have a bearing on the issue of a right to healthcare. For example, victims of asthma might reasonably claim that they have a right to clean air and that the state has a duty to guarantee a certain level of environmental regulation.

Does the extension of the scope of citizenship rights also include the idea of living forever? Can the 'everlasting citizen' emerge alongside the newly reformed sexual citizen? In the Marshallian model, there was an implicit understanding of the normal life cycle in which work, marriage, reproduction and retirement followed each other in a fairly stable and regular pattern. The deeply aged and the centenarian did not figure significantly in Marshall's scheme, since it was assumed that through savings from employment and with a modest pension, a couple might see out their (relatively short) lives without falling into poverty and dependency. All of these assumptions have been rendered obsolete by changes in the nature of work, the decline of adequate work-related pensions, high divorce rates, flexible retirement and longevity. If we try to house the rights of the geriatric subject in the mould of citizenship, we will have to rethink citizenship very profoundly.

If citizenship rights are the rights of membership in a discrete political community, human rights are those rights that are held by virtue of being human. These are typically inert and passive rights without matching duties. Human rights are often invoked by reference to victims, especially in relation to genocide. It can be said that citizenship and human rights are fundamentally different kinds of rights that should be analytically and politically kept distinct. Yet, the experience of the last fifty years has pointed in exactly the opposite direction. The concern to defend human rights has often outmatched the defence of citizenship as entitlement, status and social membership. In addition, there is increasing confusion about the differences between human and social rights of citizens. For example, in much radical literature in the United States, when sociologists argue that Americans are denied their human rights, they often talk about the inadequacies of healthcare, education and housing, but in another political culture, such inadequacies would be described as a failure of citizenship and not a failure of human rights. I want to suggest that for most citizens, human rights would be either supplementary rights or entitlements that might be claimed against the state when other measures have failed.

Citizenship is essential for cultivating civic virtues and democratic values. The notion of duty cannot be separated too sharply from rights, and this balance between right and duty, however imperfect, is the essence of citizenship. Citizenship is vital partly because when people put investments into their nation states, they can assume that they have a legitimate claim on that state when they fall ill, or become unemployed or become too old to support themselves. The past contributions to the community become the basis of legitimate claims on the commonwealth. In this respect, they can see or experience a clear connection between effort, reward and virtue. Citizenship in this way involves, often covertly, an education in civic culture in which, because citizens are patriotically proud of the society to which they belong, they are therefore committed to defending its democratic institutions. In terms of Aristotle's (1998) *Nicomachean Ethics*, citizenship creates civic virtues that can only be produced by an education in a particular political and social habitus. It is not clear what virtues flow from human rights that, following John Rawls, exist to address urgent and immediate crises such as famines resulting from failed states. By contrast, citizenship virtues emerge from the humdrum politics of everyday life in democratic societies. This is where the significance of cities for both cultivating democratic virtues in everyday politics and linking these virtues to cosmopolitan virtues becomes apparent. It is in cities as democratic spaces that 'acts of citizenship' unfold and constitute links that bind various sites of becoming citizens (Isin and Nielsen 2008). De Grey and the Immortalist movement have cut the tie between right and duty, just as they have disconnected entitlement and virtue.

I have explored some of the problems that might surround
the claim to prolongevity on the part of citizens as a social right.
These claims would have an initial plausibility, since a citizen
might claim that a government has a duty to provide for the health
and security of the members of society. On that basis, one might
say that a government has a duty to sustain the lives of its citizens
into deep old age, lives that are dignified and meaningful. One
problem that I have described is that such a right, without a
significant increase in resources and improvements in technology,
would have negative Malthusian consequences. Various changes
might be attempted to cope with this problem. The first would be
to expect the elderly to work longer into old age on the basis of
flexible retirement. The second would be to force workers to make
enhanced savings into state or private retirement funds. The third
would be to expect children to make greater contributions to their
parents' retirement needs. The fourth would be to change the basis
of pension funds through privatization. The fifth would be to
develop social policies to further reduce fertility levels. These
assumptions might be feasible if, for example, we were expecting
life expectancy to increase on average around two years every
decade, but they are not feasible in the scenario described by
de Grey and Kurzweil in which large numbers of people would
be surviving well beyond 120 years. With significant longevity,
the framework of Marshallian or welfare citizenship would break
down because there would no longer be a balance between rights
and duties, and no relationship between expectations and resources.
If we assume that, in fact, the diseases of old age could not be
entirely cured, then no welfare state, as we know it, could cope with
the demands of the deeply aged. It is claimed, for example, that
given the increase in Alzheimer's sufferers in the United States,
these care costs alone will destroy the American healthcare system
by 2030. De Grey has to make the unlikely assumption that not
only can we live very long lives, but that these can be free
of impairment and disability. We can anticipate, therefore, that as
the framework of citizenship for the elderly failed, people would
turn increasingly to some notion that they possess a human right
to live forever.

If this discussion of citizenship and social rights provides one
framework within which the prolongation of life might receive
some politico-legal justification, the other foundation for an

individual to judge his or her life would be through an aesthetic interpretation of Nietzsche. It is evident that Nietzsche's criticisms of the routinization and standardization of modern society were based on what we might call a radically aristocratic principle. Only by defying the conventions that make life meaningful for the individual can the soul achieve health. We must fashion our lives as a work of art if we are to justify our existence, and this requires the protection of a radical autonomy. Many will argue that such an ethic can have little general relevance, and yet the idea of creativity as an ideal is widespread. It occurs in particular in philosophical speculations about ageing. For example, Thomas Kirkwood (1999, 242) in *Time of Our Lives* observes that 'Freedom makes us individually responsible for our choices and actions. Is this why we readily drug ourselves into inactivity with low-demand time-fillers when we could do so much? Let us be truly alive, so that when old age finally robs us of our vitality, we may feel that the time of our lives was well spent.'

In many respects, this critical observation well captures the thrust of Nietzsche's condemnation of modern nihilism.

## Conclusion: Ethics and Scarcity

How could one reasonably assume that one's use of resources did not reduce the chances of subsequent generations to live satisfactory lives? Given global warming, it seems likely that all future generations will experience serious natural depletion and hence, will live lives that are less than optimal. Writing this study of ageing in late 2008, it is already clear that the world is facing serious shortages of water, rice, and soya bean. It is very doubtful that an elderly population could be supported without some rapid changes in food production and without confronting a Malthusian crisis. The relationship between rights and duties is becoming increasingly unbalanced. I propose, therefore, that we cannot easily solve the resource problems – overdependence on oil, the management of water supplies, and so forth – without fundamental changes to and improvements in world governance. We can, however, start thinking seriously about developing what we might call an 'ethic of longevity', namely, a set of assumptions or values that might in principle offer some ethical justification not for existence, but for life.

In this study of the problems of enhanced longevity, I have sought to distinguish between several types of question. These are (1) can we survive forever? (2) can we live forever? and finally, (3) ought we live forever? The answer to the first appears to be negative, but it is the case that we could radically extend life. Most scientists believe that de Grey's claims about rejuvenation have little support from modern science and the application of his project is impractical. In any case, survival or mere existence as such has no significant moral issues. It comes with no moral baggage. We might say, following Descartes, 'I eat, therefore I am', but this is not an ethical claim. Mere survival is not in itself virtuous, but rather a matter of luck in terms of what genetic legacy I have inherited. The struggle for longevity may be merely a product of a competitive consumer society characterized by excessive greed and individualism. By contrast, in the next chapter I want to define living as opposed to existing by the use of a metaphor from biology, namely, that to live is to avoid rigidity. It is through being flexible that one can avoid what I want half-humorously to called 'social rusting'. To live well is to avoid excessive accumulations of waste. The notion 'to live forever' means to live in such a way that life remains a journey in which there is more or less continuous self-development.

We can expand this idea by borrowing from Nietzsche who argued that the only ultimate purpose to life (as opposed to bare existence or bare life) is to 'become who we are', i.e., to develop ourselves into a work of art (Nehamas 1985). To live creatively in the world presupposes a heroic ethic. To live successfully in these terms is to avoid resentment as the basic form of nihilism (Schutte 1984). Nietzsche argued that one aspect of resentment in modern society was resentment against time itself. Such an ethic might be a valuable counterforce to pessimism in terms of Nietzsche's 'yes-saying' philosophy. The justification for life must include the notion of living life creatively and productively in order to contribute to human existence. To live life to the full in cultural terms is to leave a significant deposit that might add to human culture, making it richer and more diverse. Without such an ethic, it is difficult to see how life could be morally justified. It provides one possible criterion for departing this world, not when we are corporeally rigid, but culturally and spiritually so. In this ethic, one's life as a work of art needs to be constantly refashioned if it is to be constantly creative.

Once we cannot continue to participate in a process of self-creation, then we are no longer developing ourselves and in addition, we are no longer contributing to society. Further, assuming that de Grey's picture of prolongevity is a utopian dream, then old age will be characterized by impairment and infirmity – at least in the medium term. My argument implies that if we have a right to life, we then paradoxically have a duty to die under a variety of conditions when, for example, our continuity threatens the whole balance of justice between generations.

# Chapter Eight

## The Aesthetics of Ageing

An aged man is but a paltry thing,
A tattered coat upon a stick, unless
Soul clap its hands and sing, and louder sing
For every tatter in its mortal dress.

— W.B.Yeats,
'Sailing to Byzantium' from *The Tower*

### Introduction: Types of Survival

We can now see that the controversial but simple question – can we live forever? – has a variety of answers. In retrospect, we can now distinguish three basic forms of survival (Callahan, 2009). The first is basically the status quo, which is a relatively long life in historical terms, but with all the disability and immobility that normally goes with ageing. This scenario is obviously undesirable for the individual and costly for society in terms of rising healthcare bills. The second type would be an extension of life with little disability and a quick death. In this form, medicine has successfully addressed most of the diseases of ageing without offering us immortality. From an individual perspective, this outcome is clearly desirable. Finally, we could contemplate decelerated ageing which would simply mean slowing down the ageing process, and then there might be arrested ageing in which ageing could be delayed or deferred for an indefinite period. The aim of the Immortalists is some version of arrested ageing in which morbidity could largely be eliminated and immortality could be delivered through extensive geriatric engineering. This outcome is clearly problematic from a social and economic point of view, and it may be deeply disturbing for the individual, given the problems of boredom and despair that I have tried to describe earlier. A significant improvement in life expectancy is already taking place, and various forms of decelerated and compressed ageing look practical and feasible. Therefore, the developed societies need to create radical policies towards ageing, because the consequences of the demographic transition or secular shift, in whatever form, are far-reaching and fundamental.

The Immortalist objective is – to solve the riddle posed by the myth of Tithonus – a utopian ambition and a fantastic dream. However, we need to take the ambition and the dream seriously. Firstly, Immortalism as a programme tells us a lot about the society in which we live, especially its individualism, its fixation with technology and its unquestioning confidence in science. The dream of a long and trouble-free life tells us a lot about the rise of the Baby Boomer generation, its lasting influence and its reluctance to leave the stage. Secondly, the Immortalist programme does bring to our attention a range of exciting and imaginative aspects of medical technology and research that *may* in the long term have a radical impact on the life span. I have already suggested by reference to such figures as Lindbergh, Carrel and Barnard that much of yesterday's technological gimmickry is now commonplace. What was a fantastic dream – to fly across the Atlantic – is now routine. Barnard's brilliant heart operation is now an everyday occurrence. It would therefore be irrational to rule out the possibility that some aspect of cryonics, for example, might not be adopted by mainstream medical practice in the future. Consequently, it is prudent to attend closely to developments in nanotechnology and stem cell research to be aware of such long-term possibilities. Immortalism also brings into sharp focus the contrast between different developments of technology. For example, some techniques that are part of the longevity project – such as cosmetic surgery – have few serious social consequences. We need to guard against the development of technologies that serve individual desires and do not serve any obvious medical need, but may have unanticipated social consequences. This is the fear generated by Immortalism. Finally, the dream of immortality brings into sharp relief the whole moral problem of how any significant extension of life might be justified.

## Justification in Rights and Art

To avoid a conventional or mechanical view of ageing in the question 'Can we live forever?' I have defined living by the use of a metaphor from biology, namely that to live is to avoid rigidity. It is through being flexible that one can avoid what I have previously called 'social rusting'. To live well is to avoid excessive accumulations of useless waste. To live forever in a manner that can be justified, at the very least in aesthetic and psychological terms, means to live in such a way that life remains a journey in which there is more or less continuous self-development.

We can expand this idea of life as an aesthetic creation from the philosophy of Nietzsche, who argued that the only ultimate purpose to life (as opposed to mere existence or bare life) is to 'become who we are'. This goal involves developing ourselves, as far as we can, into a work of art. To live creatively in the world presupposes the acceptance of a heroic ethic. To live successfully in these terms is to avoid resentment and nihilism as the basic forms of negativity. Nietzsche argued that one principal example of resentment in modern life was against time itself. We should not resent the mere passage of time. Such an ethic might be a valuable counterforce to the purely medical view of living forever as simply creating the conditions whereby people could survive with a tolerable level of health or, in fact, a tolerable level of discomfort. The justification for life that we might take from Nietzsche is simply, in his terms, to live life creatively and productively in order to contribute to the health of human society by creating strong individuals. To live life to the full in social terms is to leave a legacy that might add to human culture, making it richer and more diverse. Without the development of this type of ethical position, the justification of extended life becomes problematical. It offers at least one criterion for leaving this world not when we have become moribund and morose, but when we are still culturally and spiritually lively. In such a senescent ethic, life as a work of art can be refashioned constantly and creatively. This way of looking at the problem of a creative life is unquestionably demanding and exacting, and in this sense it may be thought to be unrealistic and unreasonable, but it does bring out sharply the profound difference between mere survival and a vibrant life. The good life within this heroic ethic cannot be measured in terms of blood pressure or cholesterol.

Once we cannot continue to participate in a process of self-creation, then we are not only unable to continue to develop ourselves, we can no longer contribute to society. Further, assuming that de Grey's picture of prolongevity is a utopian dream, then old age will be characterized by impairment and infirmity. My argument implies that if we have a right to life, we then paradoxically have a duty to die when we have ceased the task of self-creation. Without this aesthetic dimension, our longevity is simply a drain on resources. In the long run, the boredom alone would kill us.

In making this distinction, I have also argued that one cannot separate the well-being of the individual from the reform of society. I have expressed this relationship between individual creativity and social reform by the somewhat unusual combination of Nietzsche and Malthus. As we have seen, Malthus was very much caught up in the debate about whether society could be improved alongside the organic improvement of human beings, and he recognized, however implicitly, that any prolongation of life would require either an increase in available land or an improvement in the productivity of labour through technological advances. He was a pessimist in the sense that he believed that neither land nor technology could ultimately improve the situation of the urban working class – he held somewhat different views of the rural working class whose lives, he assumed, were happier and healthier than industrial workers. By contrast, on the surface of it, Nietzsche does not look like a *social* philosopher. When Nietzsche did overtly address social and political questions, his attitude to the masses looks as unpromising as Malthus's attitude towards the Poor Laws and the working class. Neither could be accused of harbouring democratic values. Nietzsche's ethic is overtly aristocratic, and he condemned modern society as a place where the herd might triumph over the individual, and he therefore bemoaned the loss of a world in which genuinely heroic acts and values could survive.

Nietzsche's philosophy can therefore be adequately characterized as a 'politics of the soul' in which he saw self-development as a heroic struggle to master the instinctual life to promote the health of the individual (Thiele 1990). Consequently, Nietzsche's whole philosophy can be seen as an exploration of the problem of individualism in modern society where there is an overwhelming threat of standardization and regulation. In this respect, we can treat Nietzsche as a social thinker whose philosophy has a close relationship to the sociology of Weber in the sense that Weber also saw society as subject to an endless and ineluctable process of rationalization. In the 'iron cage' of modern society, we are all reduced to mere cogs in a machine (Turner 1996).

Is Nietzsche's philosophy just another brand of subjectivism? While Nietzsche was self-absorbed, his philosophy was aimed to awaken people to the death of God and the need to revalue life. He also craved friendship, but his journey was necessarily lonely. He recognized that 'society' was necessary for the great majority of men. Given the death of God, we are of necessity forced to think seriously about how we might live our lives without secure boundaries and directives. For Nietzsche, moral persons must to shape their lives according to their own values.

His view of life as struggle and, at its most advanced, a work of art, provides us with a model of what ageing might entail – the aim of the heroic individual is to create a well-ordered soul which has achieved a balance over emotions and desires. Every experiment has to be undertaken and every avenue has to be explored if we are to become who we are. This is the real doctrine of the overman – not the Nazi fantasy of a superman. It is in many respects the realization of Aristotle's notion of excellence or virtue. While Nietzsche did not, to my knowledge, think much about old age, he did concern himself a great deal with issues to do with food, diet, exercise and, generally, what he called 'the little things' of everyday life (Stauth and Turner 1988). The well-balanced soul also strived for a balanced health. Clearly, Nietzsche's ethic is aristocratic, or at least demanding. It could be argued that his ideal of the well-ordered soul is too demanding and too energetic to offer any real or practical guidance. Yet it is worth remembering that Nietzsche assumed that this quest for personal excellence through struggle – and especially a struggle through which the individual would experience considerable suffering – was a road strewn with failures and disappointments.

Nietzsche's overman provides a figure in whom we can make a distinction between life as mere survival and life as a creation – as an aesthetic achievement. In the end, he believed that what does not kill me in this struggle to create myself will give me strength.

Alongside this aesthetic vision, I have tried to draw attention to the fact that any extension of life must be considered alongside the reform of society. This issue of individual improvement and social reform was the important message of the social reformers around Paine, Godwin, Wollstonecraft and Condorcet. The organic perfection of 'man' had to be set in the context of a far-reaching reform of society – the abolition of the aristocracy and the monarchy, the extension of the franchise to women, the improvement of agriculture and the reform of education. Although the pessimistic criticism of the reformers often appeared to be triumphant in the writing of Burke and Bentham, social improvement in Europe and North America did take place – wages rose, famine became uncommon, women got the vote and adult literacy became more or less universal. In our day, the extension of life must also take place alongside a revival of active citizenship, the rebuilding of public institutions, the improvement in pensions and a more equitable system of taxation. However, the debate about longevity cannot be confined to nation states. We need a global strategy to deal with ageing populations, declining natural resources and global warming. My principal criticism of the Immortalist agenda is that it does not consider the engagement with the political economy debate that starts with writers like Malthus. If, from an economic point of view, scarcity is a given, where will we find the resources to sustain the deeply aged without damaging the life chances of people in developing societies and without limiting the opportunities of young people in the developed world?

## Conclusion: Individualism, Suffering and Virtue

I am sixty-four years of age. I have written this book partly because I am conscious of the huge advantages I have enjoyed by the simple fact that I was born in 1945 and enjoyed the benefits of a relatively successful welfare state. I have spent much of my adult life as an academic writing about the body, health and citizenship. My main ethical concern is that my Baby Boomer generation has made the conditions that my children face far less promising than the circumstances of my own generation. The environment is under serious threat; employment opportunities look bleak; and the world looks very unstable. Globalization has created a situation where these threats are no longer confined to certain parts of the world. While the next generation may survive longer, it is by no means clear that the quality of their lives will be superior to those of us who lived through the postwar boom and survived the Cold War. The point of this book is to establish a critique of the scientific optimism of the Immortalists, but at the same time to recognize that the quest to live longer by the application of science will proceed with or without criticism. We might hope, at least, that the criticisms of the life extension programme will generate a more realistic and effective public debate.

In my academic career I have been concerned to develop an aspect of the social sciences that now goes under the title 'the sociology of the body'. The aims of this branch of sociology have been very diverse, but one objective has been to criticize Cartesianism, which I take to be an empirical epistemology that treated the mind and body as distinct and separate. The sociology of the body has been critical of all mechanical methods of studying the human body and therefore critical of the notion that ageing was simply an engineering problem. The sociology of the body draws attention to the fact that any general solution to the ageing problem would have to address the body as a whole. Finding a cure for the ageing brain cannot take place without paying attention to the body as a whole. Compressing the speed by which the pancreas grows old has to recognize the body as a complete entity. Because we are embodied and not just a mind housed in a disposable body, solutions to the ageing problem have to address the embodied self. This fact of embodiment makes cryonics look very unpromising, because the uniqueness of the self is bound up with the uniqueness of the ways in which we are embodied. The Immortalist programme for living forever looks like an engineering strategy that ignores our embodiment and treats the body as simply a faulty vehicle of the self. In this study, I have paid close attention to the Christian idea of resurrection, because the theological debate about the body often looks more sophisticated than the modern discussion of the body.

What we might call the Lindbergh theory of the body reduces our corporeal existence and its demise to a collection of faulty pumps, levers and propellers. By contrast, Thomas does not, in the New Testament account of resurrection, quiz Jesus as to the state of his mind. He wants to put his fingers in Jesus's side. Afterwards he is reassured that this embodied person is indeed the living Christ brought back from the dead. While biological scientists have reduced life to the map of a large set of genes, we need to recognize that the human being is embodied. Their bodies do not come as merely an addendum to the person. If I am to live forever, it must be with some integrity of my whole body. A set of brilliant but disconnected engineering inventions will not give us life, but only survival, and probably anonymous survival without meaning and virtue. However, medical engineering will take place whether we like it or not. The prizes, the rewards and the investments are too great to be delayed, let alone terminated, by criticism from social scientists and theologians, but at least we should not go blindly on as if the medical utopia was not also at some level a medical nightmare.

# Bibliography

Abercrombie, Nicholas, Stephen Hill and Bryan S. Turner. 1980. *The Dominant Ideology Thesis*. London: Allen & Unwin.

Agamben, G. 1998. *Homo Sacer: Sovereign Power and Bare Life*. Stanford: Stanford University Press.

American Academy of Anti-Aging Medicine (2006) available at: http://www.worldhealth.net

Appleyard, Bryan. 2007. *How to Live Forever or Die Trying: On the New Immortality*. New York: Simon & Schuster.

Aries, Philippe. 1974. *Western Attitudes towards Death from the Middle Ages to the Present*. Baltimore and London: Marion Boyars.

Aristotle. [350] 1998. *Nicomachean Ethics*. London: Oxford University Press.

Battin, M.P. 1987. 'Age Rationing and the Just Distribution of Health Care: Is There a Duty to Die?' *Ethics* 97: 327–340.

Beck, Ulrich. 1992. *Risk Society. Towards a New Modernity*. London: Sage.

———. 2000. *What is Globalization?* Cambridge: Polity Press.

Bell, Daniel. 1987. 'The World and the United States in 2013.' *Daedalus* 116 (3), 1–31.

Berger, Peter L. 1967. *The Sacred Canopy*. Garden City, NY: Doubleday.

Berger, Peter L. and H. Kellner. 1965. 'Arnold Gehlen and the Theory of Institutions.' *Social Research* 32(1), 110–113.

Berger, Peter L. and Thomas Luckmann. 1966. *The Social Construction of Reality*. Garden City, NY: Doubleday.

Binstock, R.H. 2003. 'The War on "Anti-Aging Medicine"' *The Gerontologist* 43 (1), 4–14.

———. 2004. 'Anti-Aging Medicine and Research: A realm of Conflict and Profound Societal Implications' *Journal of Gerontology: Biological Sciences* 59A (6): 523–533.

Birmingham, Peg. 2006. *Hannah Arendt and Human Rights*. Bloomington: Indiana University Press.

Blackburn, Robin. 2002. *Banking on Death or Investing in Life: The History and Future of Pensions*. London: Verso.

Bobbio, Norberto. 2001. *Old Age and Other Essays*. Cambridge: Polity Press.

Bourdieu, Pierre. 2000. *Pascalian Meditations*. Cambridge: Polity Press.

Bourdieu, P. and L. Wacquant. 2002. *An Invitation to Reflexive Sociology*. Chicago: University of Chicago Press.

Brown, Guy. 2008. *The Living End: The Future of Death, Aging and Immortality*. London: Macmillan.

Burke, Edmund. 1955. *Reflections on the Revolution in France*. New York: The Liberal Arts Press.

Burton, Robert. 1927. *The Anatomy of Melancholy*. London: Chatto & Windus.

Bynum, Caroline Walker. 1991. *Fragmentation and Redemption: Essays on Gender and the Human Body in Medieval Religion*. New York: Zone Books.

Callahan, David. 1987. *Setting Limits: Medical Goals in an Aging Society*. New York: Simon & Schuster.

Callahan, David. 2009. 'Life Extension: Rolling the Technological Dice.'

Cheyne, George. 1724. *Essay of Health and Long Life*. Oxford: George Strahan.

———. [1733] 1976 *The English Malady*. Delmar, NY: Scholars Facsimiles & Reprint).

———. 740. *An Essay on Regimen*. London.

———. 1742. *The Natural Method of Cureing the Diseases of the Body*. tThird edition. London: George Strahan and John and Paul Knapton,.

Cole, Thomas R. 1992. *The Journey of Life: A Cultural History of Aging in America*. Cambridge: Cambridge University Press.

Comfort, A. 1956. *The Biology of Senescence*. London: Routledge & Kegan Paul.

Conners, George F. 1923. *Rejuvenation: How Steinach Makes People Young* New York: Seltzer.

Cooper, M. 2006. 'Resuscitations: Stem cells and the crisis of Old age.' *Body and Society* 12 (1), 1–23.

Cornaro, L. 1558. *Discourses on the Temperate Life*. [published as *The Art of Long Living*. New York: Springer, 2005].

Dahrendorf, Ralf. 1959. *Class and Class Conflict in an Industrial Society*. London: Routledge & Kegan Paul.

Davies, Stevan L. 1995. *Jesus the Healer: Possession, Trance and the Origins of Christianity*. London: SCM Press.

de Beauvoir, Simone. 1972. *Old Age*. London: Andre Deutsch and Weidenfeld and Nicolson.

———. 1989. *The Second Sex*. New York: Vintage.

de Condorcet, Marie Jean [1795] 1955 *Sketch for a Historical Picture of the Progress of the Human Mind*. New York Library of Ideas.

de Grey, A.D.N.J. 2003. 'The foreseeability of real anti-aging medicine: focusing the debate.' *Experimental Gerontology* 38 (9), 927–934.

———. 2004a. 'Aging, Childlessness, or Overpopulation: The future's right to choose.' *Rejuvenation Research* 7 (4), 237–238.

———. 2004b. 'Leon Kass: Quite substantially right.' *Rejuvenation Research* 7 (2), 89–91.

————. 2004c. 'Three self-evident life-extension truths.' *Rejuvenation Research* 7 (3), 165–167.

————. 2004d. 'Welcome to Rejuvenation Research.' *Rejuvenation Research* 7 (1), 1–2.

————. 2005. 'The ethical status of efforts to postpone aging: a reply to Hurlbut.' *Rejuvenation Research* 8 (3), 129–130.

de Grey, A.D.N.J., B.N. Ames, et al. 2002. 'Time to Talk SENS: Critiquing the Immutability of Human.' *Annals of the New York Academy of Sciences* 959, 452–462.

de Grey, Aubrey (with Michael Rae). 2008. *Ending Aging: The Rejuvenation Breakthroughs That Could Reverse Human Aging in Our Lifetime.* London: St Martin's Press.

DeBernardi, Jean. 2006. *Chinese Popular Religion and Spirit Mediums in Penang Malaysia.* Stanford : Stanford University Press.

Dey, Ian and Neil Fraser. 2000. 'Age-based Rationing in the Allocation of Health Care.' *Journal of Aging and Health* 12 (4), 511–537.

Dormandy, T. 1999. *The White Death: The History of Tuberculosis.* London: The Hambledon Press.

Drexler, Eric. 1986. *Engines of Creation: The Coming Era of Nanotechnology.* New York: Doubleday.

Dubos, René. 1959. *Mirage of Health: Utopias, Progress and Biological Change.* London: George Allen & Unwin.

Dumas, Alex. and Bryan S. Turner. 2006. 'Age and ageing: the social worlds of Foucault and Bourdieu' in J. L. Powell and A. Wahidin (eds.) *Foucault and Ageing.* New York: Nova Science Publishers.

Dvorsky. 2002. 'The drive to be posthuman. An exorable and necessary human imperative' available at: http://archives.betterhumans.com/Columns/Column/tabid/79/Column/319/Default.aspx

Edmunds, June and Bryan S. Turner, 2002. *Generations, Culture and Society.* Buckingham: Open University Press.

————. 2005. 'Global generations: social change in the twentieth century.' *British Journal of Sociology* 56 (4): 559–577.

Elder, Gary H. Jr. 1974. *Children of the Great Depression: Social Change in Life. Experience* Chicago: Chicago University Press.

Esping-Andersen, Gosta (with Duncan Gallie, Anton Hemerijk, and John Myers.) 2002. *Why We Need a New Welfare State.* New York: Oxford University Press.

Ewen, Stuart. 1976. *Captains of Consciousness: Advertising and the Social Roots of the Consumer Culture.* New York: McGraw-Hill.

Featherstone, Mike. 2007. *Consumer Culture and Postmodernism.* London: Sage.

Foucault, Michel. 1970. *The Order of Things.* London: Tavistock.

————. 1977. *Discipline and Punish: The Birth of the Prison.* Harmondsworth: Penguin Books.

————. 2000. 'Governmentality,' in *Power: The Essential Works 3.* London: Allen Lane, 201–222.

Friedman, David M. 2008. *The Immortalists: Charles Lindbergh, Dr. Alexis Carrel, and their Daring Quest to Live Forever.* New York: Harper Perennial.

Fries, James F. 1980. 'Aging, natural death and the compression of morbidity.' *New England Journal of Medicine* 303, 130–135.

Fukuyama, F. 2002. *Our Posthuman Future: Consequences of the Biotechnology Revolution*. New York: Farrar, Straus and Giroux.

Gehlen, Arnold. 1988. *Man: His Nature and Place in the World*. New York: Columbia University Press.

Georgescu-Roegen, N. 1971. *The Entropy Law and the Economic Process*. Cambridge, MA: Harvard University Press.

Giddens, A. 1990. *The Consequences of Modernity*. Cambridge: Polity.

Giddens, Anthony. 1999. *The Third Way: The Renewal of Social Democracy*. Cambridge: Polity.

Godwin, William. [1793] 1946. *Enquiry Concerning Political Justice, and its Influence on Morals and Happiness*. Toronto: University of Toronto Press.

Goodman, J.C. and G.L. Musgrave. 1992. *Patient Power*. Washington, DC: Cato Institute.

Gouldner, A. 1960. 'The Norm of Reciprocity: A Preliminary Statement.' *American Sociological Review* 25 (2), 161–178.

Gruman, Gerald J. 1966. 'A History of Ideas about the Prolongation of Life: The Evolution of Prolongevity Hypotheses to 1800.' *Transactions of the American Philosophical Society* 56 (9), 1–102.

Gruman, Gerald J. (ed.) 1979. *The "Fixed Period" Controversy: Prelude to Ageism (Aging and Old Age)*. New York: Arno Press

Grundy, E. 2005. 'Reciprocity in relationships: socio-economic and health influences on intergenerational exchanges between Third Age parents and their adult children in Great Britain,' *British Journal of Sociology* 56 (2), 233–255.

Harber, C. 2004. 'Life Extension and History: The Continual Search for the Fountain of Youth,' *Journal of Gerontology: Biological Sciences* 59A (6), 515–522.

Harrington, Allan. 1973. *The Immortalist: An approach to the engineering of man's divinity*. St. Albans: Panther.

Hayflick, L. 1995. *How and Why We Age*. New York: Ballantine.

———. 2000. 'The future of ageing.' *Nature* 408 (9), 267–269.

———. 2005 'Anti-Aging Medicine: Fallacies, Realities, Imperatives,' *Journal of Gerontology: Biological Sciences* 60A (10), 1228–1232.

Heidegger, Martin. 1962. *Being and Time*. Oxford: Blackwell.

———. 1977. *The Question Concerning Technology and Other Essays*. New York: Harper & Row.

———. 1995. *The Fundamental Concepts of Metaphysics*. Bloomington: Indiana University Press.

Hobbes, Thomas. 2003. *Leviathan or the Matter, Forme and Power of a Commonwealth*. London: Thoemmes Continuum.

Ignatief, Michael. 2000. *The Rights Revolution*. Toronto: Anansi.

International Longevity Center, USA. 2001. *Workshop Report: Is There an Anti-Aging Medicine?* available at: www.ilcusa.org/_lib/pdf/pr20011101.pdf

Isin, Engin F. and Greg M. Nielsen, (eds). 2008. *Acts of Citizenship*. London: Zed Books

James, William. 1922. *The Varieties of Religious Experience*. New York: Longmans, Green and Co.

Kapp, M.B. 1998. 'De facto health-care rationing by age. The law has no remedy,' *Journal of Legal Medicine* 19: 232–249.

Kass, L. 2001. 'L'Chaim and its Limits: Why Not Immortality?' *First Things* 113 (May), 17–24.

Kass, L. 2002. *Human Cloning and Dignity: The Report of the President's Council on Bioethics*. New York: Public Affairs.

Katz, Steven. 1996. *Disciplining Old Age: The Formation of Gerontological Knowledge*. Charlottesville: University of Virginia Press.

Kent, Bonnie. 2001. 'Augustine's Ethics,' in Eleonore Stump and Norman Kretzmann (eds). *The Cambridge Companion to Augustine*. Cambridge: Cambridge University Press, 205–233.

Kinsley, Michael. 2008. 'Mine is Longer than Yours.' *The New Yorker* 7 April 2008, 38–43.

Kirkwood, Thomas. 1999. *Time of Our Lives. The Science of Human Aging*. Oxford: Oxford University Press.

Kirkwood, Thomas. 2001. 'The End of Age.' BBC Reith Lecture. http://www.bbc.co.uk/radio4/reith2001/

Klinenberg, E. 2002. *Heat Wave: a Social Autopsy of Disaster in Chicago*. Chicago: University of Chicago Press.

Kotlikoff, Lawrence J. 2002. *Generational Accounting*. New York: Free Press.

Kurzweil, Ray and Terry Grossman. 2004. *Fantastic Voyage: Live Long Enough to Live Forever*. Rodale. Available at www.rodalestore.com

Laslett, Peter. (1965) *The World We Have Lost. English Society Before the Coming of Industry*, New York: Macmillan.

———. 1995. 'Necessary Knowledge: Age and Aging in the Societies of the Past,' in David L. Kertzer and Peter Laslett (eds). *Aging in the Past: Demography, Society and Old Age*. Berkeley: University of California Press, 3–77.

Latour, Bruno. 2002. 'Morality and Technology: The End of the Means.' *Theory, Culture and Society* 19 (5/6), 247–260.

MacLean, Iain and Fiona Hewitt (eds). 1994. *Condorcet: Foundations of Social Choice and Political Theory*. Aldershot: Edward Elgar.

Maddox, Brenda. 1999. *George's Ghosts. A New Life of W.B.Yeats*. London: Picador.

Malthus, Thomas Robert. [1798] 2004. *An Essay on the Principle of Population*. Oxford: Oxford University Press.

Marmor, T.R., F.L. Cook, and Scher, S. 1999 ' Social Security and the Politics of Generational Conflict,' in J.B. Williamson, E.R. Kingson and D.M. Watts-Roy (eds). *The Generational Equity Debate*. New York: Columbia University Press, 185–203.

Martin, David. 1967. *A Sociology of English Religion*. London: SCM Press.

Marx, Karl. 1963. *Early Writings*. London: C.A. Watts.

Mason, Michael. 2006. 'One for the Ages: A Prescription That May Extend Life.' *New York Times* 31 October 2006. http://www.supercentarian.com/archive/ cr.htm

Mather, Cotton. [1724] 1972. *The Angel of Bethesda*. Barre: American Antiquarian Society.

Mellor, Philip. and Chris Shilling. 1993. 'Modernity, Self-Identity and the Sequestration of Death.' *Sociology* 27 (3), 411–431.

Minkler, M. 1991. '"Generational Equity" and the New Victim Blaming,' in M. Minkler and C. Estes (eds). *Cultural Perspectives on Aging*. New York, Amityville: Baywood Press, 67–79.

Moody, H.R. 2006. 'Who's Afraid of Life Extension?' available at: http://www.hrmoody.com/art5.html

Moore, Barrington. 1970. *Reflections on Human Misery and Upon Certain Proposals to Eliminate Them*. London: Allen Lane.

Moreira, Tiago and Paolo Palladino. 2008. 'Squaring the Curve: the Anatomo-Politics of Ageing, Life and Death.' *Body & Society* 14(3), 21–47.

Mort, Frank. 1996. *Cultures of Consumption. Masculinities and Social Space in Late Twentieth-Century Britain*. London: Routledge.

Moser, K., V. Shkolnikov and D. Leon. 2005. 'World mortality 1950–2000: divergence replaces convergence from the 1980's.' *Bulletin of the World Health Organization* 83 (3), 202–209.

Nancy, Jean-Luc. 2003. *Noli Me Tangere*. Paris: Bayard.

Nederveen Pieterse, Jan. 2008. *Is there Hope for Uncle Sam?* London and New York: Zed Books.

Needham, Joseph. 1970. 'Elixir Poisoning in Medieval China,' in *Clerks and Craftsmen in China and the West*. Cambridge: Cambridge University Press, 316–339.

Nehamas, Alexander. 1985. *Nietzsche: Life as Literature*. Cambridge, Mass.: Harvard University Press.

Nietzsche, Freidrich. 1967. *On the Genealogy of Morals*. New York: Vintage.

———. 1969. *Thus Spake Zarathustra*. New York: Penguin.

———. 1972. *Beyond Good and Evil*. Penguin: New York.

Nuland, Sherwin. 2005. 'Do You Want to Live Forever?' *Technology Review*. February 2005.

Nussbaum, Martha C. 2006. *Frontiers of Justice: Disability, Nationality, Species Membership*. Cambridge, Mass.: the Belknap Press of Harvard University Press.

Olshansky, J., L. Hayflick and B.A. Carnes. 2004. 'No Truth to the Fountain of Youth.' *Scientific American* 14 (3), 98–102.

Paine, Thomas. [1791] 1995. *Rights of Man*. New York: Literary Classics of the US.

Paravicini-Bagliani, A. 2000. *The Pope's Body*. Chicago and London: University of Chicago Press.

Pearce, David. 2005. 'Interview with David Pearce: utopian biology?' *Nanoaging* December, 3–10. http.www.hedweb.com/hedethic/interview.htm

Perls, T.T. 2004. 'Anti-Aging Quackery: Human Growth Hormone and Tricks of the Trade – More Dangerous Than Ever' *Journal of Gerontology: Biological Sciences* 59A (7), 682–691.

Petersen, William. 1979. *Malthus*. London: Heinemann.

Phillipson, Chris. 1996. 'Intergenerational conflict and the welfare state: American and British perspectives,' in Alan Walker (ed). *The New Generational Contract. Intergenerational relations, old age and welfare*. London: UCL Press, 206–220.

Porter, Roy. 1997. *The Greatest Benefit to Mankind: A Medical History of Humanity from Antiquity to the Present*. Harper Collins: London.

Post, S.G. 2004. 'Establishing an Appropriate Ethical Framework: The Moral Conversation Around the Goal of Prolongevity.' *Journal of Gerontology: Biological Sciences* 59A (6), 534–539.

President's Council on Bioethics. 2003. 'Beyond Therapy: Biotechnology and the Pursuit of Happiness,' in *A Report of the President's Council on Bioethics Washington, D.C.* available at: http://www.bioethics.gov/reports/beyondtherapy/chapter6.html

Price, Richard. 1789. *A Discourse on the Love of our Country*. Reprinted in A.C. Ward. 1927. *A Miscellany of Tracts and Pamphlets*. London: Oxford University Press.

Pruit, Virginia D. and Raymond D. Pruit. 1983. 'Yeats and the Steinach Operation: A further analysis,' in Richard J. Finneran (ed). *Yeats. An Annual of Critical and Textual Studies*. Ithaca and London: Cornell University Press, 104–124.

Rabinow, Paul. 1996. 'Artificiality and Enlightenment: from Sociobiology to Biosociality,' in Paul Rabinow. *Essays on the Anthropology of Reason*. Princeton, NJ: Princeton University Press, 91–111.

Raposa, Michael L. 1999. *Boredom and the Religious Imagination*. Charlottesville: University Press of Virginia.

Rawls, John. 1971. *A Theory of Justice*. Cambridge, Mass.: The Belknap Press.

Riesman, David. 1950. *The Lonely Crowd: A Study of Changing American Character*. New York: Doubleday.

Riley, Matilda White and John W. Riley. 2000. 'Age Integration: Conceptual and Historical Background.' *The Gerontologist* 40 (3), 266–270.

Rose, Nikolas. 2001. 'The Politics of Life itself.' *Theory Culture & Society* 18 (6), 1–30.

Rush, Benjamin. 1772. *Sermons to Gentlemen Upon Temperance and Exercise*. Philadelphia: John Dunlap.

Schacht, Richard. 1983. *Nietzsche*. London: Routledge & Kegan Paul.

Scheper-Hughes, Nancy. 1992. *Death Without Weeping. The Violence of Everyday Life in Brazil*. Berkeley: University of California Press.

Schofer, E. 1999. 'The Rationalization of Science and the Scientization of Society: International Science Organizations, 1870–1995,' in J. Boli and G.M. Thomas (eds). *Constructing World Culture*. Stanford, CA: Stanford University Press.

Schopenhauer, Arthur. 2004. *On the Suffering of the World*. London: Penguin.

Schutte, Ofelia. 1984. *Beyond Nihilism.Nietzsche Without Masks*. Chicago: University of Chicago Press.

Seigel, J. 2005. *The Idea of the Self*. Cambridge: Cambridge University Press.

Shapin, S. and C. Martyn. 2000. 'How to live forever: lessons of history.' *British Journal of Medicine* 321 (23–30), 1580–1582

Shusterman, Richard. 2008. *Body Consciousness: A Philosophy of Mindfulness and Somaesthetics*. Cambridge: Cambridge University Press.

Smart, A. 2003. Reporting the dawn of the post genomic era: Who wants to live forever? *Sociology of Health and Illness* 25 (1), 24–49

Stadler, Nurit. 2006. 'Terror, Corpse Symbolism and Taboo Violation: the "Haredi Disaster Victim Identification Team in Israel."' (ZAKA), *The Journal of the Royal Anthropological Institute* 12 (4), 837–858.

Stauth, Georg and Bryan S. Turner. 1988. *Nietzsche's Dance: Resentment, Reciprocity and Resistance in Social Life*. London: Blackwell.

Stephens, Charles Asbury. 1903. *Natural Salvation, the Message of Science. Outlining the First Principles of Immortal Life on the Earth*. Norway Lake, Maine:

Stock, G. and D. Callahan. 2004. 'Point-Counterpoint: Would Doubling the Human Life Span be a Net Positive or Negative for Us Either as Individuals or as a Society.' *Journal of Gerontology: Biological Sciences* 59A (6), 554–559.

Swift, Jonathan. [1726] 2003. *Gulliver's Travels*. London: Penguin.

Thiele, L.P. 1990. *Friedrich Nietzsche and the Politics of the Soul*. Princeton: Princeton University Press.

Thomson, D. 1996. *Selfish Generations? How Welfare States Grow Old*. Cambridge: White Horse Press.

Thurow, Lester C. 1996. 'The Birth of a Revolutionary Class.' *The New York Times Magazine*, 46–47.

Trollope, Anthony. [1882] 1990. *The Fixed Period*. Ann Arbor: University of Michigan Press.

Turner, Bryan S. 1992. *Regulating Bodies. Essays in Medical Sociology*. London and New York: Routledge.

———. 2004. *The New Medical Sociology: Social forms of Health and Illness*. London: W.W. Norton & Company

———. 2006a. *Vulnerability and Human Rights*. University Park: Penn State University Press.

———. 2006b. 'The 1968 Student Revolts. The Expressive Revolution and Generational Politics,' in Alan Sica and Stephen Turner (eds). *The Disobedient Generation: Social Theorists in the Sixties*. Chicago: Chicago University Press, 272–284.

———. 2007. 'The Enclave Society: Towards a Sociology of Immobility.' *European Journal of Social Theory* 10 (2), 287–303.

———. 2008. *The Body and Society: Explorations in Social Theory*. London: Sage.

Turner, Bryan S. (ed). 1993. *Citizenship and Social Theory*. London : Sage.

Turner, Bryan S. and Chris Rojek. 2001. *Society & Culture: Principles of Scarcity and Solidarity*. London: Sage.

Turner, L. 2004. 'Life Extension Research: Health, Illness and Death.' *Health Care Analysis* 12 (2), 117–129.

Unschuld, P. U. 1985. *Medicine in China: A History of Ideas*. Berkeley: University of California Press.

van Straten, N.H. 1983. *Concepts of Health, Disease and Vitality in Traditional Chinese Society. A Psychological Interpretation*, Wiesbaden: Franz Steiner Verlag.

Veith, Ilza. 1949. *The Yellow Emperor's Classic of Internal Medicine*. Berkeley and Los Angeles: University of California Press.

Vincent, John. 2003. 'What is at stake in the 'war on anti-ageing medicine' *Ageing and Society* 23, 675–684.

———. 2006. 'Ageing Contested: Anti-ageing Science and the Cultural Constrution of Old Age.' *Sociology* 40 (4), 681–698.

Waldron, Jeremy (ed). 1987. *Nonsense Upon Stilts: Bentham, Burke and Marx on the Rights of Man*. London and New York: Methuen.

Walker, Alan. 1996. 'Intergenerational relations and the provision of welfare,' in Alan Walker (ed). *The New Generational Contract: Intergenerational Relations, Old Age and Welfare*. London: UCL Press, 10–36.

Warnock, Mary and Elisabeth MacDonald. 2008. *Easeful Death: Is There a Case for Assisted Dying?* Oxford: Oxford University Press.

Weber, Max. 1930. *The Protestant Ethic and the Spirit of Capitalism*. London: Allen & Unwin.

———. 1991. 'Science as a Vocation,' in *From Max Weber: Essays in Sociology*. London: Routledge, 129–56.

Weismann, A. 1891. *Essays Upon Hereditary and Kindred Biological Problems*. Oxford: Clarendon Press.

Williams, Bernard. 1973. *Problems of the Self: Philosophical Papers 1956–1972*. Cambridge: Cambridge University Press.

Williamson, John B., Tay K. McNamara and Stephanie A. Howling. 2003. 'Generational Equity, Generational Interdependence and the Framing of the Debate over Social Security Reform.' *Journal of Sociology and Social Welfare* 30 (3), 3–14.

Wilson, Bryan. 1966. *Religion in a Secular Society*. London: Watts.

Wollstonecraft, Mary. 1972. *Vindication of the Rights of Woman*. Harmondsworth: Penguin.

World Bank 1994. *Averting the Old Age Crisis: Policies to Protect the Old and Promote Growth*. Oxford: Oxford University Press.

World Transhumanist Association. 2006 available at: http://www.transhumanism.org.

Yeats, William Butler. 1935. *A Full Moon in March*. London: Macmillan.

———. 1938. *New Poems*. New York: Cornell University Press

———. 1939. *Last Poems*. Dublin: Cuala.

Ziegler, P. 1969. *The Black Death*. London: Collins.

Zolo, Danilo. 2001. 'The "Singapore Model": Democracy, Communication and Globalization,' in Kate Nash and Alan Scott (eds). *The Blackwell Companion to Political Sociology*. Oxford: Blackwell, 407–417.

# Index

Abrahamic religions 60
Ageing 2–5, 7–27, 29, 31, 35, 37, 39,
    41, 48, 49, 51, 52, 58–60, 63, 64,
    67, 69, 70, 73–75, 79, 80, 83, 86,
    87, 99–105, 111, 112, 115,
    117–119, 121, 124–126, 129,
    135, 139–141, 143–145
    Aesthetics of 26
    American attitudes toward 60
    As engineering problem 2, 5,
      64, 145
    As a loss of projects 25
    As inflexibility 25
    As accumulation of waste 25
    As a disease 22, 64
    As a health problem 58
    Bio-gerontological theories 10
    Body as failing machine 3, 4
    Cellular degeneration 16
    Compressed 140
    Dietary prevention of 63
    Individual 17, 73, 100
    Kirkwood theory of 18, 22, 121
    Modern theory 17
    Normal 48
    Philosophical speculations
      about 135
    Political economy of 69, 70
    Psychopathology of 24
    Radical policies towards 140
    Rate of ageing 13
    Research on 18
    Science of 22
    Sociology of 20
    Traditional framework 17
    Western medical doctrines
      about 51
Alcor 62, 63
Alzheimer's disease 15, 74, 134
America 14, 16, 28, 36, 37, 40, 57–59,
    75, 85, 131, 133, 134, 144
American Academy of Anti-Aging
    Medicine 20, 63
American attitudes toward ageing 60
Americans for Generational Equality
    (AGE) 8
Anti-ageing 3, 6, 19, 21, 73, 74
    Drugs 6
    Public discourse 21
    Science 19
    Technology 3, 21, 73, 74
Anti-Catholicism 32
Appleyard, Bryan 62, 66
Arabic alchemy 53
Aristotle 51, 133, 143
Australia 36, 76,

Baby Boomer generation 5, 38–41, 63–66, 70, 83, 104, 105, 140, 145
Bacon, Roger 51–53
Barnard, Christiaan 3, 4, 140
Beauvoir de, Simon 8, 9, 25
Beetles, The 40
Bell, Daniel 36, 37
Bentham, Jeremy 61, 131, 144
Black Death 76, 94
Blackburn, Robin 82
Blair, Tony 81, 82
   Blair-Brown years 82
   Government 81
   New Labour 81
Bobbio, Norberto 8
Britain 12, 34, 35, 40, 103–105, 130,
British Pension provisions 80
British Retirement Plans Survey 85
Brown, Guy 27, 66
Buck Institute 63
Buddhism 46, 47
Bunyan, John 58
Burke, Edmund 32, 35, 131, 144
Burton, Robert 56, 57
Bynum, Caroline 50, 96
Byron, Lord 35

Calvinism 58–60, 99
Canada 13, 76
Carlyle, Thomas 30
Carrel, Dr. Alexis 4, 19, 140
Cartesianism 5, 9, 57, 145
Cato Institute 84
Cell 19
Cheyne, George 16, 56, 57
China 5, 37, 46–49, 63, 77, 78, 95
   civilization 49
   medicine 47
   migrant labour 75
   physicians 63
Christianity 9, 12, 33, 47, 50, 53, 54, 58, 60, 61, 90, 91, 94–100, 104, 110, 113, 145, 146
   Christian duty of care toward the body 54
   Christian eschatology 50
   Christian materialism 61

Early Church 50, 54, 96
   Resurrection, ideas of 61, 97–99, 145, 146
   Second Coming 50, 96
   Slough of Despond 58
Christology 53
Clairault, Alexis 32
Clinton, Michigan 62
Cold War 40, 145
Cole, Thomas 59
Coleridge, Samuel 35
Comfort, Alex 10, 11, 17
Complete Perfection School 49
Concordat of Worms 51
Condorcet, Marquis 8, 30, 31–34, 71, 125, 144
Confucianism 46, 47
Congo 6
Conners, George 45
Cornaro, Luigi 16, 31, 55, 56, 60
Cryonics Institute 30, 60

d' Alembert, Jean le Rond 32
Dahrendorf, Ralf 76
Darwin, Charles 10, 120
Death 2, 4, 7, 8, 10–12, 14, 15, 17, 18, 22, 33, 34, 41, 47, 48, 50, 59–64, 70, 71, 73, 87, 89–91, 93–99, 102–106, 111, 112, 121, 124, 139, 143
   American attitudes toward 60
   As outcome of failed bodily machines 4
   As unacceptable 64, 70
   As pathological 73
   As normal 73
   Life after 50, 90, 91, 96–99, 103, 104
   Preventing premature 71
   Preparation for 59, 95
   Principle causes of 14, 18
Deathist 2, 29
De Grey, Aubrey 2, 3, 5, 18, 23, 34, 69, 117, 127–130, 133, 134, 136, 142
Depression 1, 85, 102–104, 124, 127
Descartes, Rene 136

Diderot 32
Dongbin, Lu 48
Drexler, Eric 62, 65
Dubois, Rene 73

Economy 21, 28, 30, 32, 35, 39, 40, 55,
    69–72, 75, 79, 82, 131, 144
    And labour migration 39, 75
    De-industrialization 79
    Global 79
    Healthy 82
    Political 28, 30, 32, 35, 39, 55,
        69–71, 131, 144
Emmons, Nathaniel 59, 60
England 13, 14, 32, 33, 58, 91, 104
    Church of 33
    England and Wales 13, 14
Engels, Frederick 35
English malady 56
Enlightenment 8, 21, 29, 32, 33, 35,
    58, 60
Eos 27
Evangelical perfectionism 60
Experimental Surgery Division 4
Extropy Institute 63

Falklands War 40
Familism 83
Field, Frank 81
Foresight Institute 65
Foucault, Michel 43, 55, 74, 91, 108
France 8, 13, 32, 40, 80
Franklin, Benjamin 60, 61
French Revolution 29, 32, 131
Freud, Sigmund 45
Friedman, Milton 79
Fries, James 15
Fukuyama, Francis 7, 20

Generation 6, 7, 10, 13, 15, 17, 22,
    23, 40, 41, 44, 58, 64, 70, 71, 73,
    75, 83–87, 93, 102–105, 117, 118,
    122, 128, 129, 135, 137, 145
    Equity (GE) 71, 83, 84
    Interdependence (GI) 84
    Intergenerational conflict 58, 70,
        71, 73, 83

Intergenerational justice 22, 23, 31,
    93, 117, 122, 128, 129, 137
    Of pensioners 84
    Of the Depression 85
    Post-war 40, 63, 105
    X 41
Germany 13, 67, 80, 81
Gerontology 2, 10, 16–19, 22, 29, 38,
    86, 92, 93, 126
    Basic presupposition of 16
    Bio-gerontology 2, 10, 19, 126
    Cellular 18
    Micro-bio gerontology 17
    New gerontology 22
    Utopian gerontology 92, 93
George, Stefan 67
Georgescu-Roegen, Nicholas 24
Giddens, Anthony 81
Girondist party 33
Gobel, Dave 64
Godwin, William 8, 30, 31, 33, 124, 144
Gray Panthers 38
Great Britain 12
Greek 27, 51, 54, 100, 113
    medical regimen 54
    mythology 27, 100
Grossman, Terry 64
Gruman, Gerald 11, 12, 20, 47
*Gulliver's Travels* 1, 69, 103

Haire, Norman 45
Han dynasty 46
Hayflick, Leonard 17, 18, 121
Hayflick Limit 18
Heidegger, Martin 22, 101, 102, 109
Herbert, George 55
Hermetic Order of the Golden
    Dawn 45
HIV/AIDS 6, 37, 70, 71
Horkheimer, Max 67
Human Genome Project 21
Hyde-Lees, Georgie 46

Immortalist 6, 7, 19, 24, 27, 29, 39,
    63, 70, 71, 73, 86, 87, 102, 105,
    106, 117, 124, 128, 133, 140,
    141, 144, 145

Immortalist (*Continued*)
   Ethos 70
   Framework 128
   Immortalism as a programme
      140, 145
   Modern 24, 63
   Paradise 87
   Social movement 6, 70, 71,
      102, 133
   World-view 7, 105
India 37, 115
Indonesia 37
Islam 60, 61, 95
Israel 60
Israeli Institute of Forensic Science 61
Italy 80

Japan 13–15, 29, 37, 69, 75, 105
Jefferson, Thomas 32
Jesuit Colleges 32
Jesus College Cambridge 33
Jewish, ultra-orthodox 60, 61
   Haredi 60, 61
John, Prester 51
Johns Hopkins University Medical
      School 86
Judaism 60, 61, 95

Kabbalah 46
Kass, Leon 20
Kennedy.J.F. 40, 104
Keynes, John Maynard 39, 40, 77
   Keynesian policies 77
Kinsley, Michael 64
Kirkwood, Thomas 17–19, 22,
      121, 135
Khrushchev, Nikkita 40
Kurzweil, Ray 30, 64, 130, 134

Labour Party (UK) 40, 80–82
   New Labour 81, 82
Laslett, Peter 12, 15, 104
Legislative Assembly 32
Leibniz 32
Leiden school of medicine 57
Lessius, Leonard 55, 56
Lindbergh, Charles 14, 19, 145

Longevity 1, 3, 11, 12, 16, 18, 19, 22,
      23, 25–29, 39, 43, 44, 46–49, 51,
      52, 55, 58–60, 63–66, 69, 71, 73,
      75, 84, 87, 92, 99, 100, 102, 106,
      116, 117, 121, 126, 127, 132,
      134–136, 140, 142, 144
   Debate 25, 37, 144
   Engineering of 19, 28
   'Ethic of longevity' 135
   Flexible retirement and 132
   For privileged generation 75
   Foundation of 49, 60
   Healthy 66
   Knowledge of 44
   Modern quest for 39, 46, 65
   Principle genes 18
   Taoist thinking of 46
   Techniques of 43, 46, 48
Luddites 2, 73
Lutheranism 55

Macmillan, Harold 40
Malaysia 15, 76
Malthus, Daniel 33
Malthus, Thomas 8, 23, 24, 28,
      30–39, 43, 70, 71, 125, 126,
      131, 134, 135, 142, 144
   Malthusian argument 34, 35
   Malthusian crisis 39, 135
   Malthusian legacy 37
   Malthusian logic 30, 126
   Malthusian pessimism 34, 39,
      125, 126
Malthusianism 31, 35, 36
Marshall, Thomas H. 132, 134
Marx, Karl 35, 76
Massachusetts Institute of
      Technology 19
Mather, Cotton 57, 60
Methuselah 60
Methuselah Foundation 63, 64
Methuselah Institute 30
Methodists 57, 59
Mexico 37
Montagnard Constitution 33
Moreira, Tiago 19
Myanmar 6, 70

Nanorex 65
Nanotechnology 5, 19, 61, 62, 64, 65, 140
NASA 65
National Insurance Act of 1946 79, 80
Necropolis 86
Needham, Joseph 47
New Testament 53, 98
New England 58, 59
New Zealand 76
Nicene Creed 50, 95, 96
Nietzsche, Friedrich 90, 92, 93, 96, 99,
    107, 111, 125, 135, 136, 141–144
Nuland, Sherwin 127
Nussbaum, Martha 35, 123

Old Testament 59
Olin Foundation 84
Osler, William 86

Paine, Tom 32, 125, 131, 144
Palladino, Paolo 19
Paravinci-Bagliani, Agostino 51, 52
Parkinson's disease 15, 74, 100
Parr, Thomas 60
Parsons, Talcott 77
Petersen, Christine 65
Philippines 37
Phillipson, Chris 83
Portugal 40
Price, Rev. Richard 32, 35
Prolongevity 11, 12, 21, 24, 27, 29, 31,
    34, 38, 47, 52, 63, 70, 92, 93, 99,
    101, 102, 104, 117, 125, 128–130,
    134, 137, 142
  Benefits of 27, 92
  Critics of 29, 130
  Discourse on 12
  Indefinite 34
  Proponents of 31
  Quest for 38, 63
  Theology of 12
Protestantism 54, 57, 95
Puritans 58, 59, 66

Reagan, Ronald 41, 86
Resources 2, 3, 6–8, 20, 22–24, 26, 28,
    30–32, 34, 39, 46, 67, 70, 72–74,

77, 83–86, 105, 106, 116–119, 122,
    124, 126, 127, 129–131, 134, 135,
    142, 144
  Distribution of 46, 83, 131
  Expenditure of 67, 118
  Natural 3, 6, 24, 70, 129, 144
  Production of, to sustain welfare
    state 77
  Redistribution of 72
  Scarce medical 73
  Social and economic 70, 126
  Struggle for 72
Rhineland capitalism 80
Ribemont, Aisne 32
Ricardo, David 24, 30, 125
Rights 3, 7, 20, 23, 24, 26, 32, 33, 35,
    70–73, 76, 77, 79, 108–114, 116,
    117, 120–135, 141
  Contributory 7, 76, 131, 132
  Health, of elderly 71
  Human 3, 20, 26, 32, 33, 70–73,
    108–111, 113, 114, 116, 121,
    123–125, 127, 129–133
  Social 76, 109, 114, 117, 120, 121,
    123–127, 131, 132, 134
Rockefeller Institute 4
Rolling Stones 41
Roman Church, early 66
Rousseau, J.-J 33
Russia 37
Russian revolution 67
Rush, Benjamin 60

Salerno medical school 51
Segni, Lothar of 51
Scarcity 6, 24, 30, 39, 72, 109, 116, 117,
    119, 120, 129, 131, 135, 144
Schumpeter, Joseph 35
Second World War 24, 77
Sen, Amartya 35, 123, 124
Sexual Reform Society 45, 48
Scottsdale, Arizona 62
Shakespeare, William 1, 89, 115
Shelley, Percy 35
Silicon Valley 63
Singapore 38, 75, 77, 78
  Central Provident Fund (CPF) 78

Singularity Institute 63
Social Security Administration 14
Southeast Asia 21
Spain 40, 93
Stephens, C.A. 31
Strategies for Engineered Negligible
    Senescence [SENS] 2, 30, 63, 127
Steinach, Eugen 44, 45
Suez crisis 40
Summers, Lawrence 79
Swift, Jonathan 1, 69, 87, 103

Taoism 46–49, 60
Technology 2–7, 21–24, 29, 31, 36,
    39, 43, 62, 66, 73, 74, 99–101,
    104, 107, 113, 116, 122, 127,
    134, 140, 142
  Anti-ageing 3, 21, 73, 74
  Biomedical 73
  Biotechnology 73
  DNA 62
  Geriatric 7
  Medical 5–7, 29, 101, 107, 113, 116,
    140
Thailand 15, 21, 37, 76
Thatcher, Mrs. 39–41, 79–83, 86
  Conservative government 80
  Years 41
Thatcherism 40
Thurow, Lester 85
Tithonus Fallacy 27, 28, 39, 41, 116
Trinity College Library 44
Trollope, Anthony 86

United Nations 26, 71, 123
United Kingdom 3, 15, 39, 76, 80,
    83, 120

Conservative and Labour
    governments 80
National Health Services 15
Office of Health Economics 15
United States 13, 14, 37–39, 58, 64,
    76, 82, 83, 133, 134
Universal Declaration of Human
    Rights 26, 71, 123, 127, 129, 130
University of London 61
University of Vienna 44, 45
Utopian 2, 7, 8, 28, 29, 34, 51, 72, 73,
    92, 93, 100, 129, 137, 140, 142
  Environment of plenty 72
  Promise of biotechnology 73
  Thought 2

Vietnam 37, 41, 104
Virgin Mary 50, 96
Voltaire 32

Walker, Alan 83, 84
Warhol, Andy 66
Warring States Period 46
Weber, Max 66, 67, 90, 99, 116, 143
Wesley, John 54, 57
Weismann, August 10, 11, 17–19, 121
Wollstonecraft, Mary 30, 35, 144
World Transhumanist
    Association 30, 63

Yeats, W.Butler 44–46, 139
Yellow Emperor 49, 50

Zolo, Danilo 77